THE GYN

Aline d'Arbrant

essay

For Valerie Solanas,
in memory of our discussions
on the benches of Central Park.

INTRODUCTION: GYNARCHY : AN UTOPIAN REALITY ?

I - A MILLENIAL AND UNIVERSAL THEORY

Man has always tried to outdo Woman. During certain periods he has even had some luck in this regard, particularly during the christian era. But from the beginning until the end of time Woman has reigned, and She will be restored. The superiority of Women is natural, known to all – even to the animals, as we shall see soon. As for the human being, who has preferred to mask reality, first as a reaction to the absolute power of the feminine, then as a way of taking jealous pleasures in ecclesiastical powers, and finally as a way to satisfy the ridiculous self-love of the male of the species, and his bruised ego, the re-conversion to Gynarchy, begun centuries ago, is in its final phase today, even if some males, in vain, reflexively try to delay it somewhat.

The absolute power of Woman, Gynarchy, is not a mere utopia, formerly established in mythic or historical times, for the happiness of all (the first part of this work). It is also a reality. But because it has always had supporters and militants convinced (the second part), it is a utopia, or an ideal society, an El Dorado, with remaining parts that we must build.. Its practices, theories, philosophy, methods of action and persuasion will be published, known and encapsulated, and applicable in practical terms (the third part), bringing happiness to the human species and giving it a real hope today for a better life and a better existence tomorrow.

II - ANIMAL LIFE : A NATURAL GYNARCHY

Gynarchy is Mother Nature's law. A consideration of the habits of several contemporary animals will provide sufficient proof of this...

We nominate, as an introduction, the Praying Mantis, whose name, in normal usage, recalls the Femme Fatale, the woman who does away with or devours the male after use. All Women, all females, are more or less Praying Mantises. Contemporary Gynarchists know this well, but it is not only this female insect which supports their thesis. In fact, many animals have chosen Gynarchy, or submit naturally to feminine rule.

A) On the Femme Fatale and the Female Devourer

In the spider family, the difference in size between the "partners" of each sex is so pronounced that most of the time the Female is likely to confuse the tiny male for her prey. Also, during the preliminaries, the latter must approach his beauty, hat in hand, lest he end up with a crushed shell.

Copulation lasts less than half a second, and it is in the male's interest to leave quickly. But often the Female, who is larger and faster, doesn't give him the chance.

B) Castration and Death: The Consequences of male Desire.

Vagina ina Dentata is not a myth used by masochists or Gynarchists in shoddy scientific arguments. In the bee family, for example, the Virgin Queen exudes an aphrodisiac perfume. This attracts the subject/slave, who comes to perform the sexual act. Then, the Queen emasculates the one who has profaned her, and castrates him. The penis snatched during this coupling stays in the queen's genitals, dead and emasculated.

C) Sexual Freedom For the Woman

Once she has laid her eggs, the Female albatross leaves her companion to care for them until they are hatched. Freed from maternal tasks, she can then mate with other males in order to better assure the survival of her line. Numerous species of birds exhibit similar behavior: thus, among rheas, kiwis, and cassowaries, the male alone takes care of building the nest, hatching the eggs and raising the young.

D) The Freudian Return Of the male To the Female Sex.

The Female bonellia (a species of marine worm) eats with the help of its tentacle. The male fixes himself there in the larval state, then inserts in it into his genital opening in order to fertilize it. He stays there until the end of his life.

Isn't this, at bottom, the unconscious sacrifice towards which all males are drawn, including the human male: the return, from adolescence, to the uterus.

One remembers Bernard Blier and little sexist cohorts in Calmos, his son's film, finishing their days in a vaginal and eschatological cavern.

E) Simian Parental Rights are Gynarchic

Humans must apply to a judge for a divorce and for custody of the children, although in the USA and in most of Europe, Women are quite properly privileged by the system; but with simians, who don't have judges, the Woman decides everything.

For orangutans, for example, the male must ask the Mother's permission merely to touch the newborns. The female baboon entrusts her baby to a male and doesn't bother with nursing. If he is slow to take up his burden, the father is generally given a serious scolding.

F) A Multi-Racial Gynarchy

Since we began with insects, we will finish with insects and with a great lesson in humility, taught to us by certain Female fireflies.

They do not worry, as certain humans do, about choosing their males exclusively from their own species. On the contrary, they know how to imitate the luminous signals emitted by their colleagues from neighboring species, so that they might attract the males of those species. But they do so not so they might use the males normally, for procreation, but rather to abuse and eat them.

Gynarchy, therefore, is a genuinely NATURAL phenomenon, favored by the Mother Goddess. And even if he thinks of himself in purely abstract spiritual terms, it has been known since Darwin that man has animal origins, and Matriarchical law is evidenced in this non-human lineage. As the past has been Gynarchic, so will be the future.

III - WOMAN IS THE FUTURE OF MAN .

The male is unable to justify himself, not even his own existence: without Woman, he is nothing. He can neither enter the world, survive there, reproduce, nor even hope to have the least happiness there.

At the moment when he finally realizes that he has taken a totally erroneous path during the centuries in which he has held the reigns of power, the moment when the world finds itself, thanks to him, at the edge of explosion or disintegration, the human male must finally abandon his part and humbly consign his destiny to his superior Sisters.

He knows he has lost. The women know they have won. The world, finally, has reason to hope. Gynarchy will save us. It alone can save the world, the planet and the human species.

And this small book wants to be the cornerstone of the magnificent edifice that
will be built.

FIRST PART :
FROM MATRIARCHAL ORIGINS TO MODERN AMAZONS
I - PRIMITIVE MATRIARCHY

Jan-Jakob Bachofen [1] is one of the first theoreticians of Matriarchy. In his works, he proved that right from the beginnings of mankind pre-historical homo sapiens lived in fear, respect and worship of Woman. Primitive male children were naturally the subjects of their Mothers. When their first desires for copulation would arise at puberty, their Mothers would give, exchange, or sell them to the Females they had chosen for them, Females who either had bought them or won them by proofs of strength or courage.

The feminine authority, instituted by Nature, induced males, right from the start, to submit to Women, to hunt and then work for them, to serve them and obey them as their natural superiors, to fear them, and to worship them like omnipotent female magicians in contact with all the divinities of the World.

The first man, a slave to Woman, was unconditionnally submissive and happy with his privileged lot. He did not think about freeing himslef from this legitimate yoke (in fact, it was not a yoke, since it was in the natural order of things). It is only as his desire for property and power grew, that he began to rebel ; and he began to free himslef from female tutelage once he became aware of woman's alterity.

Then only, the first man became a primitive man, losing in the process the natural and divine values that his Mother and female companions had taught him. Brutal strength, lust for power, and the feeling that he was above all other species brought the process to its conclusion. Man instituted the contemptible patriarchal system.

Bachofen saw Greek tragedies as expressions of the passage from primitive promiscuity and Mothers'reign, to patriarchy. This would mean that our first "culture" was conceived in the sole objective to legitimate an usurped power.

Simone de Beauvoir at the beginning of her book dedicated to the superior sex[2], seemed to condemn Bachofen's theories. However, she recognised more or less the validity of his thesis : "... children belong to their mothers' clan and bear their names ... Communal property then is passed on through women. (...) It is thus possible to consider that, from a mystical point of view, the Earth belong to women."

From time immemorial, man has sensed woman's creative power and her alterity : these two qualities of her have ensured her pre-eminence, and have pushed man to rebellion : "Being both worshipped and feared for her fecondity, being other than man et bearing the disturbing character of whatever is other, in a certain way woman held man as her dependent...[3]"

Françoise d'Eaubonne [4] (cf infra) brought positive proofs of the existence of the Amazons and of the authenticity of their thought and of the message they have conveyed to mankind. Pierre SAMUEL [5], an academic (also *cf infra*) added other elements and proposed further tracks.

The Amazons may have been, as a myth, only the persistence of the primitive matriarchal order. Historically, as can be seen in the first writings by the historian Diodorus of Sicily, they expressed a feminine resistance to patriarchal usurpation.

II - THE AMAZONS

THE MYTHS (6)- Several mythological tales or historical narratives speak about the existence of tribes of warrior women. In these tribes, males are either suppressed at birth, or, in the best of cases, mutilated, enslaved and assigned to agricultural and domestic tasks.

Diodorus of Sicily locates these tribes at the outermost western bounds of Libya[7]. He states that they were also neighbours to the Gorgons, another Amazon tribe, and a ferocious foe of theirs. The queen of the Gorgons was Medusa. The erythrean Amazons who have been traced in Ethiopia may belong to the same tribe[8].

Under the leadership of their queen Myrina, a troop of twenty thousand female warriors and thirty thousand horses conquered the Atlantid. There, they slaughtered or enslaved for life all male subjects, an event which may be the explanation for the mythological disappearance of this people : Atlant women joined the Amazons, while their males lost their identities either through genocide or permanent slavery.

We hear of another Amazon people in Greek mythology, who lived in Asia Minor and whose territory spread from the Thermodon river till the foot of the Caucasus. Their capital city was Themiscyre. Their queen Hippolytus was killed by Herakles, during his ninth labour, in order to size her belt (in effect, the belt belonged to her father, God Ares). Another queen, Penthesilea, during the siege of Troy, had Achillus madly in love with her ; this only, alas, after he had pierced her body with his sword[9]. As tradition goes, there was also a war between the Greeks and the scythian Amazons during which the victorious Amazons camped in front of Athens on a hill they dedicated to their father (hence the etymology of the current name of the hill : the Areopagus).

The same Amazons, later repelled beyond the Caucasus, established their empire between the Don and the Danube. There was the original land of the Celtic people, who, in addition to matriarchal customs, borrowed from them their traditional instrument, the bagpipe. These Amazons conquered entire countries, like Iberia and Albania. Many women in these countries, according to Marie-France Le Fel[10], joined them, and brought their husbands or brothers as slaves. Some men voluntarily placed themselves under the yoke of these fierce warriors.

Ultimately, most mythologies mention Amazons. This should justly demonstrate that it is not a myth. The celtic Fairy, the germanic Walkyria, are both Amazon magicians. The first one, on battlefields, guide men towards death, the other is able to transform herself into a witch. Both are evidently surviving or reminiscent entities from matriarchal societies[11]. Before being mythified, they were probably simple and peaceful Amazon tribes. Jacques Marcireau[12] adheres to this thesis and gives the following scientific and historical explanation :

During matriarchy, women enjoyed authority. With the advent of patriarchy, they became slaves. This turnaround did not, however, occur without fighting.

There is no doubt that woman was defeated. But some "pockets of resistance" (as we may call them), were constituted, where they remained mistresses.

Wherever they were triumphant, women constituted these feminine nations which are known under the name of Amazons.

The Amazons, in other words the states constituted by those women who rebelled against masculine authority, can only be dated to the patriarchal era. Women, wherever they were victorious, treated men derisevely, as they were treated in the rest of the world.

It is these historically vouched for "pockets of resistance" that we are going to study now.

HISTORY - The same and first scythian Amazons can be traced in the fourth century B.C.. One of their queens, Thalestris, heading an army of three hundred Amazons, came to see Alexander the Great and asked him to make her pregnant, a request which he willingly accepted[13].

In the VIIIth century A.D., Bohemian Princess Libussa's guard was composed of Amazons. When she died, they refused to subject themselves to a male authority and took refuge, under the leadership of the beautiful Wlasta, at Diewin castle, since then called "The Girls' Castle". After slaughtering the troops of the new king of Bohemia, they swiftly colonised the surrounding territories and enacted matriarchal laws, putting men under legal slavery. In the XIXth century, The Grand Larousse dictionary was thus describing them :

She published a code, the last three articles of which ruled that men were forbidden to bear arms, under penalty of death ; that they would be allowed to ride a horse only with their legs joined and dangling to the left of the horse ; that he who would dare to appear otherwise would be sentenced to death ; that men, whatever class they may belong to, had to plow and perform all the works, while women would fight for them ; that young women would choose their husbands by themselves, and that he who would regret their choice would be sentenced to death.

The king's envoy, who came to ask for their submission, was castrated and sent back to his master. Wlasta reigned for eight years, enlarging frontiers, reinstating matriarchy wherever she went. However, in the end, the duke of Bohemia got the better of the Girls of Diewin [14].

In the XVIth century, in the surroundings of the confluence of the Orenoque and the Amazon rivers, the conquistadors, saw a tribe of women warriors which frightened them and was the cause of the name of this great river. The existence of these amazonian Amazons was still vouched for in 1972 by Von Puttmaker who discovered grottoes with paintings that left no doubts about the nature of the customs of the female inhabitants : They were Lesbians. They would kidnap prisoners only to be made pregnant and would sacrifice their male children and ephemeral husbands on a kind of altar, with a small channel alongside to let blood flow out. The sound of a flute would accompany the mating ; Western indians have such bad memories of it that their women are forbidden to play the flute [15].

In the XVIIth century, an Amazon tribe was discovered in the Caucasus region (hence very close to their original territory), the Emmetches.

At the end of the XIXth century and at the beginning of the XXth, in Dahomey, the royal guard was only composed of women warriors. There were even several armies. The most dreadful, as the story goes, was one headed by the crual Agodjie, whose Amazons drank the blood of their colonial prisoners before putting them to death.

Near the kingdom of Dalmut, in Ethiopia (thus close to the territory of pre-historical Gorgons), an Amazon tribe has a reputation for extreme fierceness.

At the end of the sixities, in the XXth century, an exceptionnally clever north-american feminist, lesbian militant, Valérie SOLANAS, created S.C.U.M.[16]. This Amazon organization was rapidly banned, in view of its avowed and published goals : to castrate and enslave all males, with a plan to supress them definitively after a while and after having stocked enough semen.

S.C.U.M. however had largely enough time to conquer thousands of followers, lesbians, feminist or simple supporters of female supremacy. Today, amazon organizations - as organizations of dominant women or of or masochistic men, expand especially in the U.S.A. (Femina Society) [17] or in Europe (Gynarchy Club).

(See card : *THE WORLD FROM ANTIQUE AMAZONS UNTIL NOW.*)

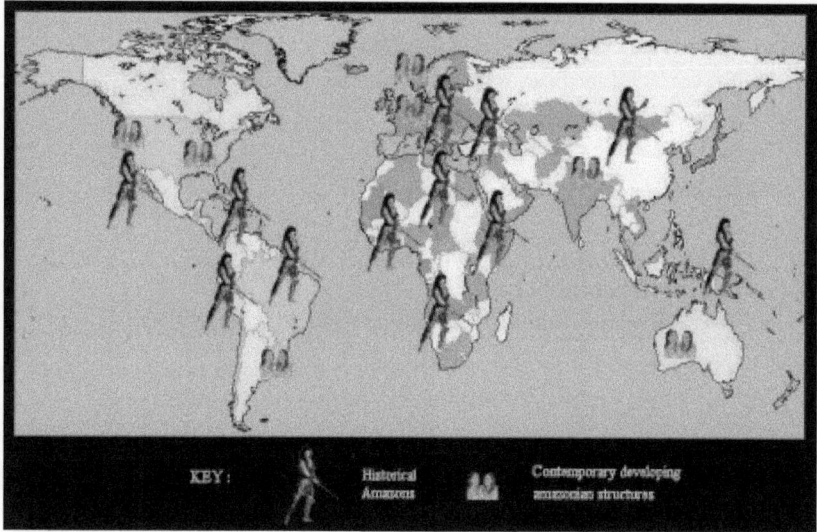

SYMBOLISM - As mentioned hereabove, mythical Amazons are a resurgence of primitive matriarchal societies. According to Paul Diel, they would be the symbol of women-who-kill men : they want to substitute men, compete with them by fighting, instead of complementing them.

This seems too rapid an analysis. It seems preferable to follow Jacques Marcireau's historical explanation mentioned previously (18), and the thesis of the Dictionnaire des Littératures, for which they symbolise the open resistance by matriarchy. [19]

In any case, according to the same source, it is the Amazons who passed on to the Catholic church their gesture of blessing (raised thumb, forefinger and middle finger) and to the French royalty, their emblem (the lily).*Amazones dans le monde :*

LEGENDE :

1 : Amazons of Scythia (Hippolyte, Penthesilea), protohistorical.

2 : Amazons of Libya (Myrina), prehistorical.

3 : *Gorgons* of Erythrea (Medusa), prehistorical.

4 : Amazons of Carpats (Thalestris), century IV.

5 : The *Girls* of Bohemoa (Wlasta), century IX.

6 : Amazons of Orenoque, century XV.

7 : Amazons of New World, centuries XVI.

8 : Amazons of California (Califia), century XV.

9 : Warrior Women of Dahomey (Agodjié), end of century XIX.

10 : Warrior Women of New-Guinea, middle of century XX.

⇢ : Possible Amazons' migration.

A : Developing Amazons' structure during centuries XX and XXI.

III - FROM SUFFRAGETTES TO WOMEN'S LIB

From time immemorial, from the Amazons up to Dominique Voynet, there have been some women who contended their intrinsic need of independence, of socio-political pre-eminence and their intellectual superiority. But it is truly in the XVIIth century that this gynarchic trend asserted itself. Then was the time of the cultural reign of Madeleine de Scudéry, Marie de Sévigné, Marie-Madeleine de La Fayette, all of whom were infinitely more cultured and intelligent than their brothers, lovers or husbands, and of the political reigns of Catherin of Russia and Christin of Sweden [20], more powerful and wiser than most of their contemporaries.

In the XVIIIth century, king Louis XVth himself gave an example of a "French Gynarchy" by choosing a Mistress who dominated France while dominating him [21]. In turn Mrs de Prie, Mrs de Mailly, Mrs de Châteauneuf, Mrs de Pompadour, Mrs du Barry govern Louis XVth ; there is hardly a minister who does not have his female mastermind [22]. At the eve of the revolution, Charles COLLE writes, about women, that "they have got such an upper hand over the French, they have subjugated them so much, that the French can only think and feel after them".

But it is indeed in the XIXth century that this "long march" by women began, a march which will probably reach its goal as soon as the beginning of the XXIst century. Women even enjoyed support by some enlightened males : positivist Comte imposed the worshipping of Woman by the people in the temple of Humankind, Prosper ENFANTIN [23] expected from a Woman-Messiah the advent of a better world and his Companions of Woman embarked to the Orient

17

looking for this Woman-Saviour who looks quite like our future Gynarchist Sovereign. Eugénie NIBOYER published la Voix des Femmes (Women's Voice). George SAND advocated free love. Flora TRISTAN believed the people would be redempted through Woman. All of this lead up to the suffragist fights of the beginning of the XXth century.

In 1903 in England, Emmeline PANKHURST created the Woman Social and Political Union, the ancestor to all our current feminist movements, and organised marches towards the Parliament and other locations. Often using provocation and violence, her suffragettes would partially win their case in the end, but after long struggles.

(See diagram : *Gynarchist Evolution of Society* in the next part.)

Thereafter, towards the middle of the century, drawing their inspiration from Emmeline's fight, Women's Lib in the U.S.A. and M.L.F. (Movement for Woman's Liberation) in France were created. Kate MILLET [24] wrote her Politique du mâle in 1970 and Valérie SOLANAS, a visionary gynarchist lesbian, founded her Society for Cutting Up Men [25] (S.C.U.M.) the following year. At last, true Gynarchy was on its way.

IV - MATRIARCHAL SURVIVALS IN THE TWENTIETH CENTURY

Some other feminine behaviours have become ever more fashionable during the twentieth century, in particular in industrialised countries. They are similar to Amazonism or Matriarchy, and probably derive their origins from these. Polyandry in particular has made a strong fashionable come-back.

In effect, Women used to content themselves, during the male chauvinistic and obscurantist centuries, with cuckolding their husbands and/or having them accept the presence (in their houses or in the matrimonial beds) of their lovers or suiters. Nowadays, they more and more choose, sometimes after a revealing divorce, to resource to polyandry and have their choices accepted by their multiple, often submissive, partners [26]. Dozens of males submit themselves to these feminine, perfectly natural demands, and do so with pleasure and gratitude. For them also these demands are very gratifying.

They know that they are not alone in being allowed to give pleasure to their Mistresses (in both meanings of the word), however they derive pride and satisfaction from that situation. Pride because it all proves that their Mistress is a desirable Woman. Satisfaction, because they feel better giving pleasure to a superior Woman for a long period of time, than to take a short pleasure from a non-gynarchist woman.

The success of the excellent book by Wanda WEBB [27], which advocates women to exploit the intrinsically masochistic tendencies in males, is a proof that the world is moving towards a universal, irreversible Gynocracy.

Progressive Women chosing this way of life are growing more numerous, and sometimes group themselves (some however prefer solitude and anonymity, and choose to live their dominant polyandry on a free lance basis) in gynarchist organizations that help them efficiently to constitute a male harem. Many gynarchist Ladies join private clubs, etc.

The future, even in the short term, belong to them ...

SECOND PART: FEMINISM, LESBIANISM AND GYNARCHY

I - THE FIRST GINARCHIST PHILOSOPHERS

We don't possess any truly Gynarchistes texts previous to the Middle Ages in spite of the certainties that we have of the high level of knowledge of some matriarchal civilizations (as the one of the Etruscans) and of the learning of some uterine or spiritual Girls of the Amazon (of Sappho in Libussa of Bohemia, the list would be long). The transmission of the theories and systems intellectual, social etc. granting the pre-eminence to the Woman was transmitted by the oral way. Weren't the provincial troubadours, militating in favor of the polite life style, the submissiveness to the Lady, which was not anything else than a Gynarchiste rule delicately renamed romantic love, at the same time the putative successors of the Roman speaker, Feminist before their time, who harangued their colleagues on the Forum about Women, and, especially talented itinerant and submissive puppets, the brokers of a mysterious medieval Feminine Gynarchist philosophy which they distributed as much as possible to the castles and the villages?

Cornelius Agrippa [28], was one of the rare Gynarchist philosophers of the Renaissance whose work survived. Indeed, in the enlightened times of the Matriarchal proto-history, it did not seem useful to develop a Feminine hegemony, since it went from oneself. Following the male rebellion which was to triumph long before the Christian era, the new patriarchal religions, to impose the masculine authority, used strength, censorship and the violence jointly [29].

One remembers the terrifying repression provoked by the revolt of the Amazons of Bohemia in the Middle Ages [30]. AT this time the Women, having neither printing nor monks (or slaves) copyists to distribute their Gynarchistes ideas (that they lost besides very quickly) and to make known their thirst for emancipation, could only take up weapons, as Wlasta, or, when they were sufficiently powerful, to elect polite " writers " [31] to recover the power that had been theirs lawfully. But, since the end of the 1500s, Women quickly realized the power of Gutenberg's invention and attempted to use it to their profit. And the men themselves, when they wanted to be pleasing to some important sovereign, had to offer them the texts celebrating their pre-eminence.

Thus, it was for **Marguerite of Austria** [32] that the philosopher Cornelius Agrippa wrote, in 1509, his Gynarchiste opus explicitly titled: *"The Superiority of Women"* [33].

To prove this Feminine superiority irrefutably, he included, in his work, subtitled "medicated Opuscule of the nobility and the excellence of the Feminine sex, and of Her superiority to the masculine", used the arguments and examples pulled from religion, the natural sciences and liberal arts. We will only make here a very fast summary, non-exhaustive, of his main arguments that used all of the resources of all known sciences, then, of course, connoted very strongly and determined religiously:

The ETYMOLOGY, from the start returns Adam to the earth and Eve to life [34]. furthermore Adam is born of a clay ball come who knows where, whereas Eve, is born of life herself.

THE most elementary THEOLOGY attests that the Creator always, during the Creation of the World, would go from the simplest to the most complex [35], from the ugly to the beautiful, from the raw to finished it, from imbecility to intelligence. Naturally the Womyn was created long after the man, only after the Creator had realized the intrinsic imperfection of Her first human creature. It was necessary that She create the Womyn so that God at last judges Her creative task finished. The Womyn is therefore the ultimate of the creatures, the crown and the end of the Creation, the perfect coronation of the set of the works of the Great architect She is the perfection of the universe (36).

GEOGRAPHY designates the Womyn again as privileged since Her creation. If the fallow fields were sufficient for the man, God preferred to create the Woman inside some Terrestrial Paradise.

The biblical HISTORY attests that most Kings and some Prophets voluntarily place one or several Womyn above the other and of themselves [37]. And are we ourselves not spellbound by the characters Judith's (who decapitated Holopherne after having seduced him), of Athalie (who took alone the power), of Salomé (who used Her charm to get the head of the Baptist), and by so many other marvelous Womyn that the Bible itself praises [38]?

THE NATURAL SCIENCES add contributions also to this demonstrating that the Feminine body is infinitely more complete and complex than that of the man. It alone prepares the fetus and alone generates the child. Her genital and sexual organs are infinitely more complete than that of the man [39]. Finally, the Womyn is more resistant to pain and lives much longer than the male of the species.

PSYCHOLOGY, PARAPSYCHOLOGY AND MAGIC also attests to the Feminine superiority. Virtue and modesty are assets of Womyn and these are the same Womyn who make the best Prophetesses and Sibyls.

PHILOSOPHY is not only a science where Womyn excel [40] but where they have the advantage, in case of an impossible failure, to be able to dominate the philosopher himself by their natural and intrinsic ability of seduction, as testified to by the myth of Xantippe riding the enslaved philosopher.

Finally, after a diatribe in opposition to the false male philosophers inhibited by patriarchal morals, Cornelius Agrippa concludes:

To finish and to summarize as briefly as possible, I affirm that it is high time for us to recognize and to proclaim the superiority of the Feminine sex: I affirm it superior in consideration of the etymology, of the natural order of the things, of geography, of the reports that the examination of the matter invites us to establish and I affirm it superior because of the examples gathered by me from religion, the natural sciences and liberal arts. All these proofs, as well as the support of the reason and the testimony of a lot of authors, drove me to discern that God has, in all domains, offered to the Womyn more of dignity and more of quality that to the men.

Other philosophers also added their contributions, sometimes modest, sometimes brilliant, to the development of the conceptual theory of Gynarchy :

Guillaume Postel, has at the same time, announce the arrival of a new Eve, Almighty, that will regenerate human kind. Won't this new Eve be made our first Gynarchist President?

Marguerite de Valois, in her learned and subtle speech asserts high and strong, in opposition to all official dogmas of the time, that there is something well divine in the Womyn.

Marguerite de Navarre (1492-1549), essentially seeking the honor and happiness of Womyn, extols the chastity and the submissiveness of Her lover to his Lady. Aren't these not the golden rules that the male correctly integrated to the system of Gynarchy must follow ?

II - LESBIANS IN THE BATTLE

Lesbians not only felt immediately concerned by the Feminist fight and its inescapable outcome, Gynarcy, but they took here and there, more and more, an active part. There was Valérie SOLANAS, one of the modern Amazons, of which we already spoke and to which we will come back, the Gouineses Rouges, in Paris, in the sixties... Today most Womyn Gynarchisteses confess some saphiques tendencies, as well as on the contrary most Lesbians militate in favor of the absolute power of the Womyn. Incontestably, the future of the World depends on Lesbians.

SAPHISM, GYNARCHY AND LESBOCRACY

Intense and fantastic is the saphic pleasure... Tirésias, who had lived as a Womyn confirmed it by the myth: if pleasure was divided in ten parts, the Womyn would have nine and the man only one of it. Not only is the male not able to, naturally and essentially, know the Feminine pleasure, or even to approach its himself, but he would be even incapable of even imagining it. Then, he can only be fascinated most of the time by the Lesbians, to resign himself to admire and be jealous of them, on the frozen pages of male "magazines", and to spend his life dreaming of being admitted, one way or the other, by a Feminine couple.

As for the Womyn, She is drawn to Saphisme by its natural appeal, by disgust for the male or by curiosity, and doesn't feel the necessity to inform the man of the stupendous and infinite pleasure that She feels with one or several other Womyn, nor has She the desire to have him share it. It is why most Lesbians exclude the male completely from the intimate life of the couple that they form.

However, they give up at the same stroke the advantages thus that they could have from this fascination that they exercise on the inferior man. A lot of groups young or more experienced, understood this however and became the dominators of males [41], Mistresses, happy and satisfied in a life where they taste the transcendent pleasures of Lesbian loves and at the same time to the joys of Feminine domination [42].

Thus, little by little, as we already know, men accept, or even search for, the yoke of the Womyn, and the Gynarchy is established. At the same time, and more and more, Womyn convert to Saphisme or, at least, no longer consider the male anymore as their only sexual partner. In the long term therefore, these are the Lesbians who are going to seize Power and govern the World.

Must one consider this future and likely Lesbocratie as a threat for the heterosexual Gynarchy that we defend, or as a desirable community ideal, or as the inescapable conclusion of the evolutionary process of human society?

Humanity was at first matriarchal. Then the males, motivated by their natural vices that the Womyn had only identified badly or not acknowledged, contested their superiority and they seized power [43], probably by strength and by the fact of their numbers (the polyandry natural of the human species encouraging this disproportion).

It is this brutal takeover that caused the creation of the nations of Amazons, that were originally that of the Womyn who revolted against the male oppression. The man can never bring an end to these " resistant " Womyn. When he succeeded in defeating a tribe of Amazons, a new one created itself. When a nation of Womyn was decimated, there always remained some survivors to carry the matriarchal message of hope for Womyn elsewhere. The men attempted by all means [44] to fight this Feminine will to regain Her natural rights. He nearly succeeded.

But it is precisely when his victory seemed completely assured, in the beginning of the twentieth century, that the " war of the sexes " resumed and that the male power vacillated, soon, to topple inexorably. It started with the suffragettes, in the beginning of the century, then by the Feminism of the sixties and the extremist movements that it generated (the Gouines Rouges, the Witches [45], the S.C.U.M. [46]) nearly all were enlivened by Lesbian fundamentalists [47]. Then, little by little, the domineering, the gynarchists and some Womyn, independent of all ideology, started surpassing the man and to dominate him or to advantageously replace him.

The man therefore begins to tremble and fear for his power. His reactions to this movement, to the pace of the irresistible tidal wave are different according to his cultures and characters. Some defend themselves, as previously, provoking the Amazon, while attempting by all means to keep his archaic prerogatives (as in the case of the religious fundamentalists of all types, of the supposedly domineering that one finds haunting, without much success, the screens of the pink minitel, of the homosexuals who prefer to remain with men to give themselves the impression of not being dominated by Womyn). Many cannot internalize this distress of the male structures and, abdicating completely, deliver himself to alcohol, to drugs, or to suicide. Others, fortunately, assume their defeat and, either become masochists (often delivering themselves temporarily into the hands of a professional Dominatrix, to receive the moral humiliations and the physical tortures that they know natural and indispensable to their male condition), or reasonably, give themselves body and soul to dominant Womyn or let themselves be enslaved voluntarily by one of them. These reasonable men, who are increasing to a phenomenal degree, become, or look to become, a Womyn's slave, or the slave of a Lesbian couple.

Here we are, in the history of Gynarchy, but are forced to note that nothing is finished. First because the Womyn's victory, although inescapable, is not yet completely assured. Secondly because this new liberty of the Womyn (although older historically) is in great peril from the males who carries in him the seeds of totalitarianism.

Indeed, when man will finally be subdued and Womyn's independence and hegemony finally made real, nothing will stop Her from discerning the extent of Her power and the total global possibilities She has acquired.

First, on the socio-cultural level: why grant some liberty to the one that has, more or less voluntarily, renounced it, who is very content being deprived of it, and that history demonstrates is incapable of using it without abusing it to some extent? It is important then, not to let the male assume even to the least degree any power. But how to get to this ultimate state? The Womyn's only alternatives: the pure and simple elimination of the males [48] or, less extreme, their rigorous physical and psychological transformation, to create an irreversible race of slaves out of them, conditioned completely to serve Womyn and never to question their state of being as such.

Then, on the psychological plan, one is able reasonably to believe that once the man is reduced to a state of slavery, and is happy with his fate, the Womyn will be content with using him solely as a servant and producer of consumable commodities. The temptation to abuse will come fatally and a lot of dominant Womyn of today succumbed this already. Soon, each Womyn will need a domestic slave AND a financial slave, then a sexual slave AND a scapegoat, etc., as soon as She feels the desire for it. It is one of the main virtues, the Womyn creates the possibilities. So each Womyn will become a small domestic, polyandrous Sovereign either to a single sexual partner, or to the head of a small team of male slaves. Then, as Her life is transformed as regards to Her comfort and well being, Her creativity, Her intelligence and Her energy are likely to be perfected again.

Finally, on the sexual plane, as one saw previously, Womyn, since they will have the right to it, will taste all sexual pleasures, and, sooner or later, those of Lesbianism also [49]. All will become then inevitably adepts of Saphisme and experts in Her so Feminine and so gratifying Arts [50] as regards to physical enjoyment. After just a few months practice of saphiques, She will be able to compare the very ordinary level of happiness that comes from copulating with a degenerate slave, and the intoxicating and magic, interminable and delectable enjoyment, felt equally and voluptuously between a Sister's arms, a refined, member of the same dominant and cultivated class of the Gynarchic Society, sharing the same pleasures, possessing the same Feminine body, the same desires, and searching for the same ecstasies. Obviously, Womyn will become the main, if not total, desired sexual companions of each other, only finding between themselves the pleasures, the feelings and the heart and the body that can give them full pleasure. For the Dominant Lesbians, the man - slave will lose therefore quickly and irreparably all sexual interest [51] and love interest (because of having lost all of his dignity).

The reigning Lesbian society (considering the total sexual, psychological and socio-cultural inferiority of the male) will consequently not allow his free or unsupervised existence. Accordingly he will effectively only exist to serve the Lesbian Community (doing productive work, domestic service, tool parent, object of distraction, etc.). Certainly, there is some fear of extremist abuses (those who favor the extermination of males) but, the in the Lesbocracy or Gynarchy the sovereigns of the world will be above all Womyn and will know how to decide therefore rationally and efficiently on what status to grant to their male inferiors.

As the revolutionary Mensheviks let themselves be overthrown by the Bolshevik extremists, the domineering Gynarchists will be supplanted (but quite to the contrary without violence) by the extremist Lesbocrates. This will imply, undoubtedly, a rapid assimilation, legal and factual, of the human males with the other animals of creation and their use as such, in accordance with their rudimentary possibilities, by the Lesbians who will have accepted them in their livestock.

(See below ble of the evolution of the Gynarchic Society)

Little by little, the male's visceral desire for reproduction and sexual pleasure will merge itself with the periodic grants of semen in the laboratories of fertilization or with the periodic drafts of seed that the discriminating Lesbian Mistresses will probably allow. The private slaves, of individual Womyn [52], will forget quite quickly that another sexual pleasure can exist other than the one to which ONLY the Lesbians reach. They will learn how to derive pleasure only through the satisfaction of their Mistresses. And the Lesbocrate world will seem quickly ideal to them, as is proved already by the fascination that all males have towards Lesbian love.

Gynarchist Evolution of Society :

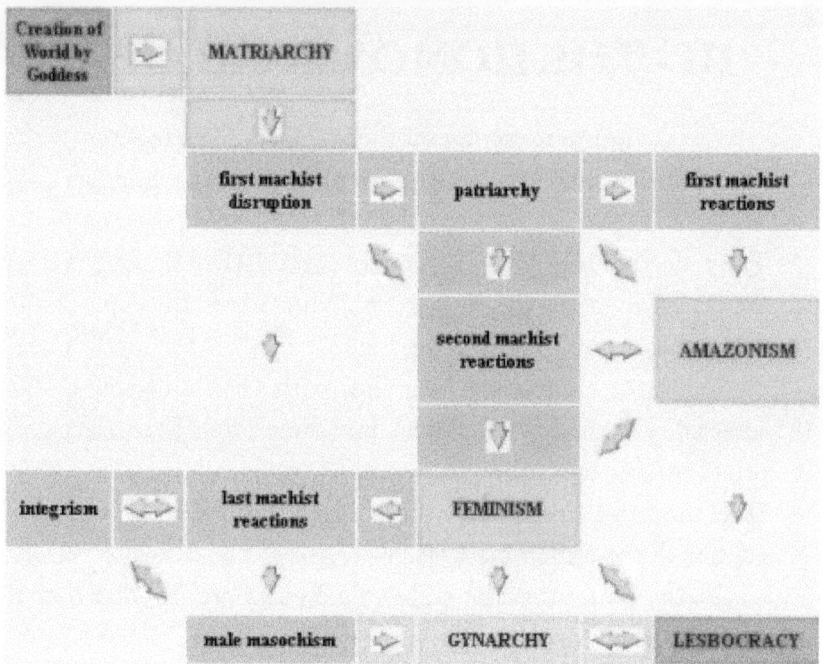

III - THE HOMOSEXUALOPHILY,

or the attraction for the inverse homosexuality,
first subconscious element of Gynarchiste thought.
" \l 2

The reflection that follows came to us precisely following this report, that each can make without particular difficulties: the appeal more and more obvious of Youth for the homosexuals of the opposite sex. The nightclubs of homosexuals overflow with Grrls and young Womyn, sometimes themselves Lesbians, but most often heterosexual, being proud to be the confidantes and close friends of these deviants. Sometimes, they justify themselves merely by confessing " to really " feel good with these effeminate males.

In the same way, the clubs of Lesbians are invaded literally by supposedly curious males, presenting themselves as " voyeurs " or, more honestly, as " masochists ". Some Womyn's clubs must literally put up barriers to these intruders to be able to satisfy their true clientele.

But the major motivations of these Grrls liking to be surrounded with false Womyn and men awkwardly trying to evolve toward the Feminine ideal, are not the same as those of these spellbound vile or obsequious men, fascinated by the physical and moral fullness exemplified by the adepts, of the Divine Sappho.

THESIS 1: The Womyn is attracted by the homosexual because of his obvious desire to imitate Her.

To be a homosexual, is before all to want to be a Womyn, or, at least, to want to resemble Her and to imitate Her. Even the act of " homosexuality " of the males is therefore a desire to appropriate the Feminine sex object, the man, and a jealous desire to substitute for the Womyn. Passive or active, the male homosexual assumes or represses his resentment at not being a Womyn and, in all cases does everything that is in his power to be accepted ", existentially and transcendentally, by Her.

The result, very naturally, is that the Womyn, in the midst of them, feels, beloved, respected and, otherwise wanted and envied. A man's homosexuality unconsciously proves to the Womyn Her psycho - sexual superiority and, being in the presence of these males who assume their inferiority by this deviation from nature, She enjoys generally strongly, and not without a certain sadism, this envious and admiring proximity.

THESIS 2: Lesbians attract the man irresistibly because of the incontestable proof that they give him of his intrinsic inferiority.

It is not only for the male about satisfying his deep desire to attend a aesthetic and imaginary romp érotico-saphiques, but to volunteer themselves for a real and violent psycho - sexual humiliation. Greatly tinted of incipient masochism, his apparent desire to take part in a Lesbian couple's lovemaking, is nearly always accompanied with a lot of obvious fantasies, such as being tied up or restrained, verbal humiliations and punishments of a more or less sever nature, etc., all of which of course he is the object of on behalf of these superior and Almighty Lesbians. From there to become aware of his visceral desire to be enslaved completely by these Womyn, there is only a step that the male generally has to take and most often does very quickly.

THESIS 3: According to Freud, Womyn and male humans all have in them, in a more or less developed way, an attraction for their own sex and a subsequent fascination for the homosexuals of opposite sex.

Some already acknowledge it; others suppress it, and some finally live it. For Womyn, in general, the consequence first is more or less a progressive disgust for the male and they opt little by little either for Lesbianism, or for relations of Gynarchic Domination of the male, or for a compromise of the two. As for the men, in most cases, they know this fascination that they feel. The " so-called " men's newspapers are more or less full of erotic Saphic images (never pornographic when there are only Womyn in them). Some males know the reasons for this bewitchment of which they are victims and veil their eyes. Others ignore it but feel attracted inexorably by all examples of Saphisme and, little by little, by those of the masculine masochism. Fortunately, a lot of males know how to draw their true findings from this latent emotional state. They go to Womyn, the true ones, that are Lesbian, and Domineering or a Lesbian couple, and offer themselves to them, as escort, submissive husband, hireling or devoted slave.

CONCLUSION: The Gynarchic feeling is intrinsic to human thought, as much in the Womyn as in the male.

It is obvious to any human being, even male, who analyzed his homosexual tendencies a little bit, if one will forgive us this neological barbarism of which we made our title, that the unconscious Gynarchic feeling, little by little guessed and than assumed, is the real motive for this apparently incomprehensible behavior. It is not necessary to be ashamed of this fascination therefore that each one feels for the homosexuals of the opposite sex but, on the contrary, to recognize it, to justify it and to strengthen it in this necessary and fundamental outcome that is the first true conversion to the Gynarchic life style and the practical application of Feminine Supremacy to daily life.

IV - THE MODERN CURRENTS OF THE FEMINIST THOUGHT.

In the last third of the 20th century, except in the countries dominated by Islam Gynarchic thought and action have little by little replaced the traditional Feminist movements. In modern Gynarchic philosophy, one essentially distinguishes three currents of thought that, by way of intellectual clarification, we qualified as: mystic - spiritual, socio-political and practical/sensual. Quite evidently, these three schools are each interdependent and are not able to sustain themselves without one another. However, we are forced to note that the contemporary intellectual thought about the origin of these dedicate themselves in general to one only of the aspects of the system that we recommend. This, unfortunately, is to the detriment of a global conception of Gynarchy that would reconcile the knowledge and the philosophically action as well as the theorizing for the betterment of the social, spiritual and the sensuality of the Womyn [58].

A) The mystical - spiritual Gynarchy.

Several Churches gather those that believe that spirituality is a necessary path for the return to Matriarchy and not, on the contrary, its outcome. However, all Gynarchists have in common the firm belief in the supreme spirituality of the Womyn, in opposition to the materialistic (or even animalism) intrinsic to Her lower fellow, and the very intriguing and educational character of the daily exercise of Gynarchic rituals. It is in the United States that one finds the largest number of Gynarchic Churches.

- The *SM church*, of San Francisco is the main Gynarchic organization in Californian. In a specific manner, it combines interest in the erotic Feminine Domination with related ideas on the worship of Womyn and the development of associated spiritual rituals. The religious services there look like the Christian rituals but are dedicated to Goddess's worship. Those that receive communion must kneel and must be hit on the shoulders and the head with a whip, as symbol of purification [59].

- The members of the *Femina-Society*, very active in all domains, define themselves as Matriarco - Feminist by nature and see the true Domination/submission as a quadruple path: physical, emotional, intellectual and spiritual. They believe that these four elements are necessary to the authentic practice of Feminine Authority.

In its spiritual goals, the Femina-Society instituted rituals of renouncement, atonement and submissiveness, organized according to the natural cycles of the Earth. The third point of its fundamental doctrine is very explicit: " *Recognition of the real Feminine Authority while following the Path of the Goddess embodied in the illuminated Femininity* ".

In France too one finds the stammering of some Gynarchistes groups with spiritual aims.

- The *Church of Jesus Scourged* has for its goal " *the schooling and the domination of the men, our inferiors, in their having to suffer to reach the divine perfection. It is a Christian Church, based on the Domination by Womyn, as the Divine* " creatures privileged of God . After a period of obedience to the Priestesses assigned to direct it, the supporter must undergo a seminary of initiation that will make it a disciple of Mistress Monique, head Priestess of the cult.

- The *Gynarchique Order of the East* gives itself for an objective " *to awaken the spiritual conscience of the Feminine aspect of Divinity through a processes of masculine devotion and suitable erotic rituals* ". Its doctrine is " *the discipline of the expiatory to surrender to the Feminine aspect of the Divinity* ". All Womyn there are welcome that are testing the path of Feminine Supremacy or are simple sympathizers. In the Temple of the O.G.E. the Mistresses and their assistants do the training in the rituals by using their available devotees. Several programs aim at " *the surrender of the devotees to the Feminine Superiority by the progressive increasing in the capacities of their tolerance,* " are proposed to the supporters in a progressive order.

B) The socio-political Gynarchy.

For most taking as a starting point **Valerie SOLANAS** and S.C.U.M. [60], the intellectuals who enroll in the ongoing socio-politic Gynarchic movement are only rarely implied on the public stage. One knows those that made know their ideas through the intermediary of a brilliant deed, of a novel of fiction extolling the Feminine Superiority or of the biography of one of the innumerable Womyn having more or less worked for Gynarchy, such as Christine of Sweden or Wlasta of Bohème. The others work anonymously, directing in the shadows of one or two men, sometimes very near to the political power, that they enslaved and converted to Feminine Superiority.

- **Marie-France LE FEL**, in Her Small historic and convenient Dictionary of the domination and the sadism of the Womyn [61], draws up an exhaustive list of these Womyn, historic or romantic, on which the present and future generations should take example to build the best world that the Gynarchists will bring to birth.

- **Marika MORESKI**, that is probably only the pseudonym of the previous, is the author of fiction novels [62] that put on stage Womyn really living daily the Gynarchic life. These novels prove undoubtedly that the gynarchists hold the truth and the key of happiness.

- Many authors, such as **Norman SPINRAD**, **Robert BLOCH**, **Robert MERLE**, **Daniel-Yves CHANBERT**, etc., under pretext of " science-fiction " (that doesn't deceive anybody) put in pages various descriptions of the ideal Gynarchic society.

- **Gini GRAHAM-SCOTT**, American, with already two works that are dedicated to this [63], contributes to the knowledge of the practices of Feminine Domination and the rites of sado-masochism that, very certainly, bring a large number of males, up to this point hesitant and nervous, to make the big step, giving back body and soul to the hands of a superior Womyn, a Mistress or an Association of Gynarchists.

- Finally, let's recall that the *Femina-Society* doesn't disregard the political aspect of our philosophy, as the points 5 to 8 of its program prove:

« *5) International promotion of the understanding of Authentic Feminine Authority as opposed to the S/M of prostitution and to the " realization of fantasies ". Our programs and publications reflect this goal.*

6) Recognition that the economic and social currents of our society are controlled financially by the males, who exclude Womyn from the government of our lives in an oppressive way. The Femina Society recognizes the need of Womyn to be sustained by males until the Feminine Sex possesses the instruments and the social support to create their own economic state. This masculine support must not dictate on no account the Feminine conduct.

7) Institution of programs, on a small or a large scale, offering service of some profit socially to Womyn in difficulties, in an effort to help elevate the statute of Womyn.

8) Considering that centuries of patriarchy cannot be overtaken without, the recognition of the necessity and the need of instituting change. We consider that the patriarchy must be :

a) neutralized through the Feminine authority,

b) shown as the destructive power it is,

c) de-activated as an instrument of oppression/destruction. »

C) The hédo - pragmatic Gynarchy.

Under this explicit neologism, we wanted to arrange all those that militate in favor of an immediate satisfaction of the legitimate Feminine requirements and that, by their example or their writings, attempt to convince the few Womyn still under the psychological domination of one or several males, or even of one of these criminal patriarchal religions, yet on their way to extinction [64]. This fight is not to disregard, but on the contrary, it is often thanks to a selfish hedonism that Womyn approach Gynarchic thought before embracing it. And it is again more often because of a young Womyn searching for Her exclusive pleasure that the male, decreased, humiliated but strangely satisfied because he was used like object or servant by the one that he wants. Note the intrinsic desire that he has for the submissive role and the excellence of the Mistress/slave relationship that Gynarchy extols.

- **Wanda Webb**, a rich American free and smart, wanted to propose the principle of the right of Womyn to train and use submissive men, or those men susceptible to become so (that is to say all), to their profit. Her pamphlet, Of the good use of the masochists [65], first defends this theory [66] and gives the results of it then [67]. Since its release, the work of Wanda WEBB has had a considerable success. Several daring Womyn considered this text like a manifesto, told us its publisher, also created good number of " farms " of slaves through all U.S.A. and even elsewhere.

- **Sophie Dompierre**, more pragmatically but with logic and experience, achieved, in a fundamental and incontestable work for all those that wish to institute a real domestic Gynarchy in their home [68], propose a real method of domination of the males.

It would be tedious (and useless, since she distributed it extensively) to summarize it here. Only specify that Sophie Dompierre reserves a whole chapter on the strategy to adopt with regard to the males who are non volunteers and, after three other very well documented parts on the various punishments, torments and necessary immobilization's to the schooling of these males, a last chapter full of ideas and good advice on " a slave's " daily use.

- **Astride** is a Militant Gynarchist, whose views are directed toward the different techniques of servitude of the male but without forgetting to explain the philosophies and the psychological justifications for it. Thus, Astride gives several reports giving, thanks to the Feminine body it self, for its ability to subdue the male. One will read, among others with interest, the three following works [69] : Power of the underskirt, The art of the excretion, the art of the suffocation [70].

This arbitrary division of the various contemporary Gynarchists tendencies into three classes (mystic - spiritual, socio-politic and hédo - pragmatic) has a goal merely to clarify and educate. Globally, all schools have a common philosophy and common practices but it was necessary, to better understand every sensitivity to proceed to this fast tour of the horizon of contemporary Gynarchist thought, before entering into a much more pragmatic survey of the methods and programs proposed by those that want to short or long term, restore the Matriarchy.

THIRD PART: METHODS OF FEMININE DOMINATION AND ACCESS TO THE POWER

The feminine superiority, today universally recognized, brought humanity, during these last years, to reconsider the paradigm of our Society completely. Thus, all psychologists, sociologists and intellectual not recovered by the male chauvinism in place recognize the absolute necessity to confide to the Womyn completely both the domestic power and the political power.

The Woman, psychologically, physically, genetically and mentally superior to the man, must today reorganize the world around her necessary pre-eminence. The hour is not to equivocations anymore and the male must immediately abandon his last bastions of influence to the Woman.

All this, of course, must begin by a renovation, as well, alas, of the feminine minds as, necessarily, of the masculine mentalities.

I - EDUCATION AND PEDAGOGY

EPISTEMOLOGY - One of the domains that were most quickly conquered by Womyn was naturally the one of education. However this forces us to note that the equality recommended in school is justified least of all when it imposes the same education on Girls and boys.

It is completely absurd to place Girls and boys in the same classes and at the same age! What a Girl understands in some days it can take a fourth of the term for the boy to assimilate. Just as the young Girl discovers the world, it beauties and its ugliness, the boy is learning to play billiards and discuss soccer. When the teenager encounters problems of sexuality, the boy wonders why he has erections. And when the young Womyn is ready to enter in to the social and active life, the boy still late to mature masturbates while looking at Girls and disregarding his work.)

This is why it is vital for our good social health and for our future Feminine Institutions not to thwart the harmonious psychological and intellectual development of Girls by putting them in classes where the cretinism of the males will level, undoubtedly towards the bottom, their superior capacities.

Is this to say that it is necessary to avoid co-education classes? Certainly, a class composed only of Girls will always be infinitely more productive and mentally efficient than all mixed classes as they are conceived of today in our schools and colleges. However researchers think that the unmethodical masculine energy, currently disruptive and ominous to the studies of Girls, could be cannibalized and used as a subordinate support for feminine education.

Thus boys of all ages could transcend their school activities while working for the main goal of the intellectual blossoming and cultural development of the Girls in their classes. In this way they would collaborate in the success of those whose incontestable intellectual superiority makes of them their natural underlings. By this method they will probably approach more nearly the feminine intelligence, without of course, ever being able to reach it.

ne of domains that was the most quickly conquered by the Woman was naturally the one of the education. However, force is us to note that the laic equality recommended in school, if it is justified incontestably socially and ethnically, the East at all when she imposes one same education to Girls and boys!

The advent of a real and definitive Gynarchy will be created by the institution of a specific teachinghe advent of a real and definitive Gynarchy evidently passes by the institution of a specific Teaching [71] and therefore by the foundation of a Gynocratic School. The creation of a school institution compliant to our ideal has proved to be absolutely necessary.

One could have considered a strict separation (disciplinary and geographical) to the teachings to each sex. But this method doesn't stand up to analysis. The male needs to be dominated by the Female from the youngest age (hence the verb "To Mother") and Girls need to learn very early to use their power, including in the school setting. This is why we chose the co-educational system for out Establishment.

It shows great promise in the face of the problem immediately raised by this choice. A great number of parents are delighted to see their Girls learning to dominate domestically, to direct socially and to govern, though less accept the idea of letting their boys learn submissiveness and the manual labor to which we educate them. There again, the analysis is bad. It is better to learn some less noble profession well and to know without difficulty how to submit to a superior Feminine will than for the male to spend his life unemployed with a submissive and banal woman as alas many now do.

(See below the first French Inscription Form for I.M.E.G.)

FICHE D'INSCRIPTION

ETUDIANTE   ou APPRENANT (1)

NOM :   NOM :
                                              Prénom :
Prénoms :   AGE :

Date de naissance :   DISPOSITIONS (1):
Lieu de naissance :
                                              - ménage
Adresse des parents :   - vaisselle
                                              - lessive
                                              - cuisine
Adresse Personnelle :   - service
                                              - secrétariat
                                              - jardinage
GOUTS :   - bricolage
     Littéraires :
                                              - AUTRES (2):
     Artistiques :   .

     Culinaires :   .

Autres centres d'intérêt :   (1)   Rayer   les
                                              mentions inutiles.
                                              (2) Préciser.

CADRE RESERVE A L'I.M.E.G. NOTES:	TRIM 1	TRIM 2	TRIM 3
DEGRE DE SCOLARITE :			
- Filles			
- Jeunes Filles			
- Adolescentes			
- Jeunes Femmes			

NOM ET PRENOM DE L'ETUDIANTE-TITULAIRE (ou de l'adjuvant):

AUTORISATION DES PARENTS : Je, soussigné(e),....................
demeurant à :...

  - autorise ma fille .... à épouser et/ou employer
l'adjuvant agréé par l'I.M.E.G. qu'elle aura choisi.

  - délègue à l'I.M.E.G., et/ou à l'Etudiante-Titulaire choisie
par elle, tous mes pouvoirs parentaux sur mon fils ....

SIGNATURES :

Men conscious of their natural inferiority and their inabilities that today search with perseverance for a "Mistress" know what happiness would have been theirs if the opportunity to enter into one of our Mixed Institutes of Gynocratic Education (I.M.E.G.) had been offered to them. But, especially in families of modest means, one finds nevertheless, parents preferring the security that our Institution offers to the risks of the traditional teaching of the state in as much as the cost of the education and residency are much lower for boys [72].

To mark the different functions inside the Gynocratic class [73], it was necessary to name the Girl, the main object of the general education, and the boy differently. For him the name "student/auxiliary" refers to his double functions: we will use the term ADJUTENT for his functions of school and personal assistant to the Girls and the one of his learning and other school activities.

As for the Girl, dedicated almost completely to studies, we will name Her logically "STUDENT" and won't add the TITULAR term to Her title that designates the part that relates to Her supervisory activities in Her dealings with boys, in particular with Her regular adjuvant. Gynarchist thought, open to ideological enrichment, creates this vision of the subordinate involvement of boys to the education of Girls. This is how the founding idea of I.M.E.G. came into being.

PEDAGOGY - For a long time researchers sequenced the educational methods arbitrarily in three convenient of basis:

1) the masterly method (the Mistress, holder of the Knowledge, transmits this one directly to the pupil),

2) the active method (the pupil, under the Mistress's direction, be going to search for himself his/her/its Knowledge),

3) the programmed method (the relation Mistress-raises is suppressed to preserve a relation, in general computer, between the pupil and the Knowledge.

One had the habit to schematize these old methods thus :

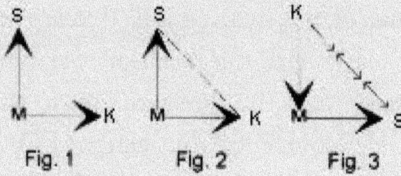

Fig. 1 - Masterly method
Fig. 2 - Active method
Fig. 3 - Programmed method

M = Mistress, S = Student, K = Knowledge, A = Adjuvant

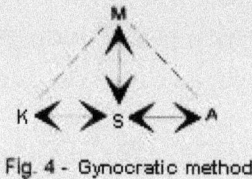

Fig. 4 - Gynocratic method

Evidently each of these three methods was in contradiction with the other two. It was necessary to wait for the first theories on Gynarchc education so that one will give up the pupil's E station in the old method and as a matter of course develop and permit relationships between each points of the triangle and thus all the senses.[74]

This is how is developed the notion of third-learning, doubling our old triangle symmetrically and allowing E, the student (in opposition to A, learning, all students of one same Mistress M distributing the same K knowledge) to be in total and permanent contact with all parts of the educational sequence.

This symmetrical triangular relationship makes itself, as indicated in figure #4 the biggest profit to E that sees the clear access to the three facets of the act of M's teaching, S and A and then achieves therefore without negative aspect the global educational function. M also keep Her access. Only A has a contact by mediator S.

48 ALINE D'ARBRANT

The perfect working of the method will develop itself therefore so that M, the Mistress, source to the E station, the student who can happily and regularly assimilate the three accesses to the educational realization, and inversely, source to the station TO learning in a position of inferiority or intellectual difficulty that will bring a double profit of a masterly educational situation in his case, since he undergoes the influence there of the Mistress and the Student.

The division in sections of ages and levels makes itself naturally on the basis of the student's physical and intellectual development, faster than the one of the learning male. The task of the male is therefore in the first place to learn well in what period of the Feminine process of maturation the student is to which he has been attached and to adapt his behavior accordingly.

Comparative Figure of Pedagogic Methods				
	Masterly	Programmed	Active	GYNOCRATIC
S > K Student direct access to Knowledge	NO	NO	YES	YES
K > S Knowledge given without intermediate	NO	YES	YES	YES
S > M Possible recourse to Mistress	YES	NO	NO	YES
M > S Intellectual contribution of Mistress	YES	NO	NO	YES
A > S A access to S Knowledge	NO	NO	NO	YES
S > A S in charge of A activities	NO	NO	NO	YES

The phase of educational intervention of the I.M.E.G. begins roughly in the student's eleventh year to finish towards Her eighteenth year. One distinguishes four natural groupings of a Student to the audient: 11/12 years, 13/14 years, 15/16 years, 17/18 years. Classes are spread therefore into two years to the maximum but can be reduced substantially according to every individual progression. The experience provided to a really motivated Girl, incoming to the institution at 12 years, can easily, with the help of an older adjuvant correctly educated, can get involved in the social and active life by Her sixteenth year.

Some months in one of the intermediate courses (Teenage Girls) are sufficient to a brilliant Student sometimes to assimilate knowledge of the program. This is not evidently the case for the apprentices. When these enter the I.M.E.G. it is imperative that whatever his age at admission, to follow the specific masculine formation to every Feminine level of education. He must understand that all boys can be made attendant to a student of any age from 11 years up.

The logical progression of the Feminine education in the institution (Girls ± Teenage Girls ± Adolescents ± Young Womyn) doesn't apply naturally to adjuvants [75]. A young male of 12 years age newly admitted to the I.M.E.G. can very well start his education as the adjuvant of a Student of the course of age "young Womyn" of age 18 years old. Requirements legitimate his Student-titular will have a beneficial effect on his understanding of the Feminine authority. In the same way, and older adjuvant, even legally an adult, because he would only give modest satisfaction or because he would have entered the I.M.E.G. late, could see himself assigned to a Student0titular of the course "Girls", six or seven years younger than him in order to have him discover the reality of the total Feminine authority.

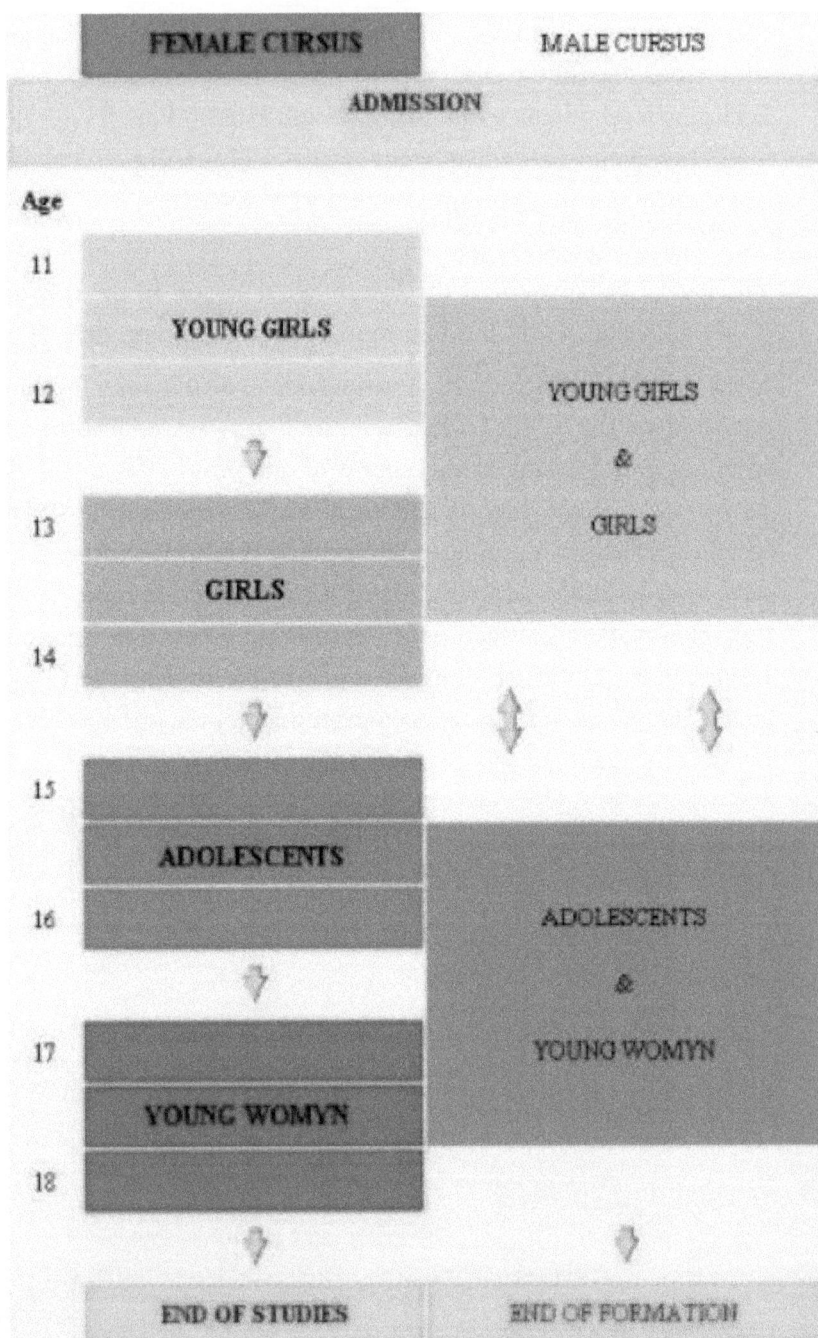

FEMALE CURSUS	MALE CURSUS
ADMISSION	

Age		
11	YOUNG GIRLS	
12		YOUNG GIRLS
13	GIRLS	&
		GIRLS
14		
15	ADOLESCENTS	
16		ADOLESCENTS
17		&
	YOUNG WOMYN	YOUNG WOMYN
18		
	END OF STUDIES	END OF FORMATION

The ASSESSMENT of Students is made in a continuous notation (grading) of 5 levels (ABCDE) in every matter including those of specific courses. The NOTATION of adjuvants is made every quarter in four areas (to 11 levels of 0 to 10) :

1 – note for the control of the Specific Course.

2 – note of faculty to the Gynocratic Auxiliary

3 – note for Course.

4 – External Service note[76].

ORGANIZATION -The Mistress faces the Students. She is thus better able to converse with them and to observe their reactions, as in the masterly method, and to complement the data that the Students have acquired through computer research and study on their own. In addition She can better observe the actions and gestures of the adjuvants since they sit behind the Students that they are assigned to. Adjuvants don't have the right to speak in class. They must take all the notes and the instructions of their Student-titular.

All the documentation is placed in the back of the course room. One finds there the closet of software, the shelves of dictionaries, encyclopedias and various books that are necessary to the research of the Students. A general, Basic Culture Library, completes this mini-research center.

Students arrange, with their adjuvants, an individual personal data processing complex at a P. C. terminal of the I.M.E.G. School. They can, during the course, use all of the computer and human material that is put at their disposition by the institution.

The classroom consists of 25 tables: the Mistress's desk, the twelve desks of Students, with returns supporting the keyboard and the monitor of their computer and the twelve worktables of the adjuvants. To facilitate Her work on the computer or Her adjuvant, the Student-titular arranges a leather armchair so that She can comfortably rotate it to work at the keyboard or turn to give some instructions to Her adjuvant.

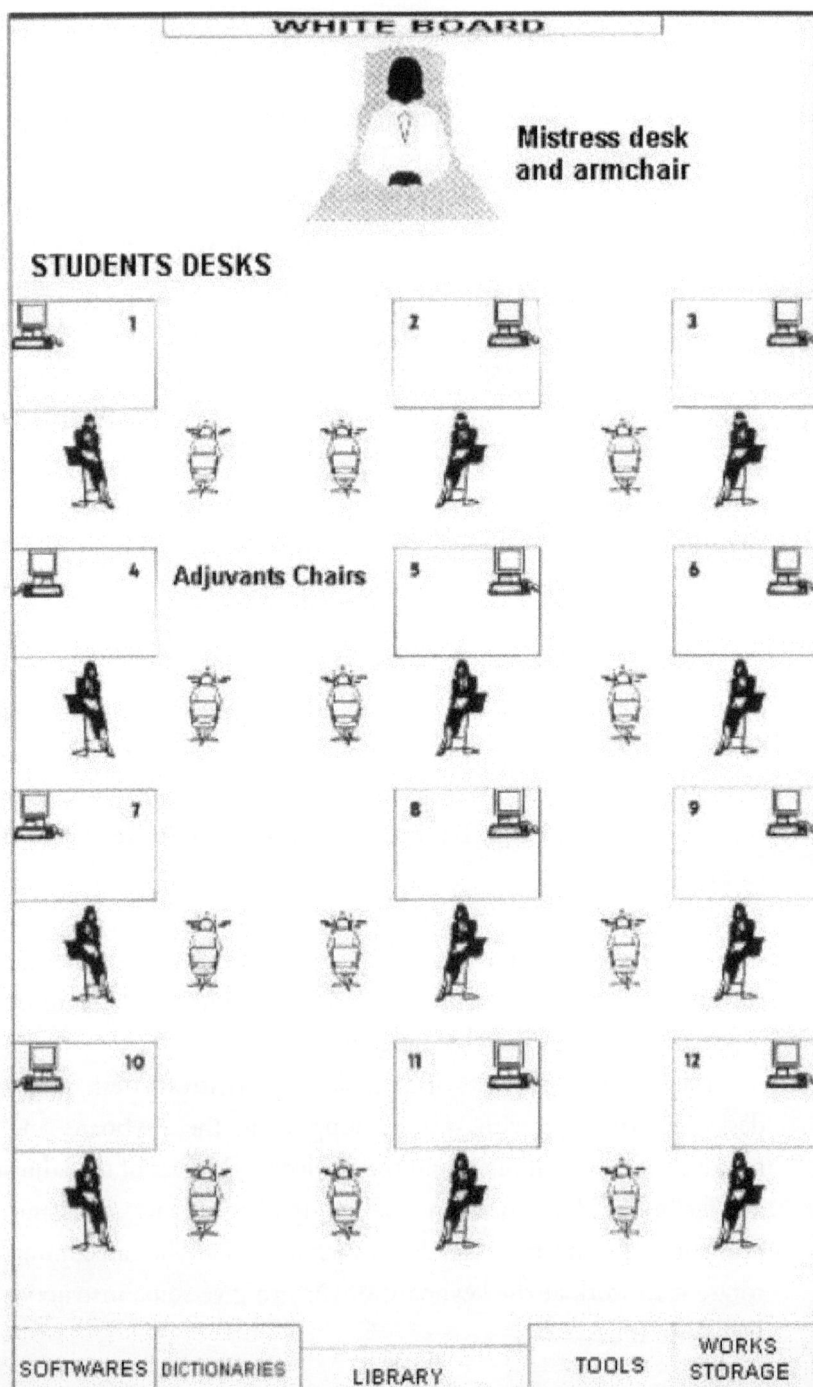

WHITE BOARD

Mistress desk
and armchair

STUDENTS DESKS

1

2

3

4   Adjuvants Chairs   5

6

7

8

9

10

11

12

SOFTWARES | DICTIONARIES | LIBRARY | TOOLS | WORKS STORAGE

2 2 222222222222222222

The small square tables, without draws, of the adjuvants are placed along the isles so that they can very quickly, fulfill the demands of their Student-titular, to reach the shelves and closets of the room and bring back as quickly as possible the required documentation. adjuvants sitting on small stools without files so that their work of copying and their frequent movements take place without noise or hindrance for the class [77].

The adjuvant and his small piece of work furniture must be placed along the isle therefore and functionally, slightly behind the student-titular to be able to observe Her needs better and, possibly, signs that She is likely to make to transmit Her orders. Placed thus, the adjuvant can remain attentive just as well to the Mistress's requirements as well as his immediate hierarchical superior.

Plan type d'un I.M.E.G.

The TIMETABLE is unchangeable, in the I.M.E.G.; in particularly for the adjuvants that must make sure that all the domestic services are accomplished with no false excuses tolerated. For Mistresses and Students, the institution allows a larger indulgence.

Mistresses give 6 courses of 50 minutes per day, therefore 5 hours in all, which leaves them ample time to prepare. Their day starts with the Feminine Specific Course, that allows them to organize the day with the help of Students, and ends with the masculine specific course, in which imperfections due to the long workday can be allowed for and the frayed nerves of the Mistress can find an easy outlet.

Students have days of 14 hours, which alternate between classes (a little less than 5 hours), sports (about 2 hours required), free time (nearly 3 hours), one hour of survey and relaxation (a little more than one hour of television).

The day of adjuvants is a little longer but doesn't reach 17 hour. If they rise earlier and go to bed later due to their various services (breakfast, the morning dishes, and interview in the Student lounge in the evening), they have enough rest times distributed throughout the day however. They have the same number of hours of courses that the Students have and a half-hour of survey besides that to compensate the intrinsic awkwardness of their sex.

The schedule at I.M.E.G. is therefore most harmonious (*see the chronological synopsis*).

06 30			Corridors Cleaning
07 00			Bathroom and WC Cleaning
07 30			Classes Cleaning
08 00		AWAKENING	Kitchen
08 30		BREAKFAST	Service
08 45			Breakfast
09 00	Class SP	LESSON SP	Students Bedrooms Cleaning
09 50			Rest
10 00	Lesson M1	LESSON M1	Lesson M1
10 50	Lesson M2	LESSON M2	Lesson M2
11 40			Kitchen
12 30		MEAL	Service
13 00			Meal
13 15			Dishes
13 45			Rest
14 00	Lesson M3	LESSON M3	Lesson M3
14 50	Lesson M4	LESSON M4	Lesson M4
15 40		SPORTS	Rest
16 00	Lesson SP		Lesson SP
17 30		STUDY	Activities by groups (garden, laundry, shoes cleaning...)
18 30			Kitchen
19 00		MEAL	Service
19 30			Meal
19 45			Dishes
20 30		TV	Study
22 00		BEDTIME	Sitting Room Cleaning
22 15			Rest
22 30			Bedtime

CONTAINS OF TEACHINGS - The general courses are essentially centered on the Students general culture (practice in three living languages of which the Maternal language is one), world affairs,

General Literature, Arts (painting, music, dance, film...), History and Geography of the World, The Sciences (math, biology, physics, etc.). In addition and advanced survey of techniques of modern management and organization, in particular by means of data processing computing. The Student will be placed to the maximum extent possible in real situations of supervising (computer and network research) and managing of personal subordinates of all ages, [78] (personal adjuvant and the global male cohort of the I.M.E.G. [79]).

Thus all conditions for the Student's total success, once She exits the institution are united both on the professional plane (general culture, scientific and technological knowledge) and in personal terms (character formed for the domination of the male underling, the psychology of command and technical expertise [80], etc...).

One hour is reserved each day to the Feminine or masculine specific teaching. It would be quite unreasonable, in the mixed residency of a Gynocratic institution, not to economize to make a distinctive education to each sex. That is why at the start of each day the Mistresses teach only the Students, without their usual male adjuvants [81], and, at the end of the day with the adjuvants without their Student-titular [82].

The adjuvant learns from the earliest age from the I.M.E.G. Student to accustom him to Her future functions of command, to teach him in thought and action (philosophically and pragmatically) the reasons for Her superior and naturally higher position in society and in short, to prepare him mentally for the jobs that the male faults oblige him to assume.

The boy, must learn quickly the domestic and servile tasks that will be his from the time of his entrance into the I.M.E.G. and thereafter, in life. One must immediately explain to him the reasons for his natural inferiority, to make him discover the truth of Gynarchy and to convince him completely of the necessity for a universal Gynarchy. The certainty of the Feminine superiority and the knowledge of his own deficiencies will help him in his tasks of being an aid to the Womyn. Not only must the young adjuvant learn very early his real functions of domestic and manual auxiliary in society to a Feminine predominance but again he must be satisfied and execute the subordinate tasks imposed by his superiors with joy and satisfaction.

DISCIPLINE – Students can organize their hours of liberty as they chose and can benefit from all recreational, sports and cultural structures of the institute. Every young Girl of the I.M.E.G. at the time of Her registration has assigned to Herself a personal adjuvant, chosen from among the masculine students, if possible of Her age, whose main mission is to attend to Her during classes and in Her life of residency. She becomes "Student-titular" to him and can use him to solve all lowly material problems of Her daily life. Thus the daily household chores of the particular room of each Student-titular is the duty of Her personal adjuvant as is the taking of notes during classes and the writing (under Her direction) of school papers.

Students have at their disposal a laundry and shoe repair shop, both situated on the male side of the establishment where they can give to their adjuvants the job of cleaning their dirty cloths and shine their shoes. The Students are not required to show any deference towards the adjuvants of whom they require these services. All students of the I.M.E.G. have to right to make a complaint to the Council of Mistresses against any adjuvant who might have caused Her a problem or embarrassed Her in any way.

Meals are served at regular hours by the cohort of adjuvants (breakfast at 8:30 AM, Lunch Noon to 12:30 and Dinner at 7 PM) and they must avoid disrupting the life of the institution by delays or recriminations without foundation. All complaints must be for cause and the Student must carry out Herself the sentence that the Mistresses will have pronounced upon the offending adjuvant. Their access to the kitchen, the launderette and the shoe repair store must be reduced to the strict minimum.

Students must learn by heart and respect to the letter the schedule that is communicated to them the day of their admission to the I.M.E.G. As soon as he learns the identity of the Student-titular under whose authority he placed, temporarily or permanently, he must as quickly as possible surrender to Her and inquire as to what She requires of him and conform accordingly.

Learning this he must take complete charge of the care of the particular room and bathroom of the Student to whom he is attached and in the same way, during hours of classes, he must make the best notes that She asks him to take and to search quickly and silently for all the documentation of which She may have need. He will very carefully write down all of the duties, which She will dictate to him. All adjuvants must naturally execute all tasks required by his Student-titular whatever they are. Besides his plain of service to his Student-titular, the adjuvant must execute the collective masculine tasks of the institution every day: cleaning of the common part of the household, the soiled cloths, preparation and service of the Student meals and by rotation service in the Laundry, Shoe repair and Vegetable Garden.

In manifest cases of abuse or incontestable bad treatment at the hands of a Student, the adjuvant can go to complain hierarchically to his Student-titular then, if litigation persists, to refer an exceptional case to a Mistress. He must know however that this last recourse can turn against him so that harm is given to him and he will be required in this case to undergo himself, at the hands of the one of which he complained, the sternest corporal punishments.

The Director of the I.M.E.G., the four main Mistresses and Student-delegates of every class, constitute the Council of Mistresses, the only authority authorized to reward and to punish. It acts at the end of each year on the promotion to higher classes and on orientation and to give to Students and students their graduation from the institution. It arbitrates, litigates and decides some disciplinary sanctions. These are to the number of eight.

Three to the consideration of Students: the warning, the blame and the exclusion,

Five to the consideration of adjuvants: the slap, the spanking [83], the flogging, the isolation [84] and the transfer [85].

With such an educational analysis, of rigorous formative rules and a project of education of this wealth, one has a system of Gynocratic schooling finally bringing a serious answer to the stagnation and the present delirium of our current governing pedagogues.

II - METHODOLOGY AND SEMANTICS OF FEMALE DOMINATION

Why combine these two apparently unrelated terms in the title of a study of gynarchic techniques? Because from the beginning it has seemed that a great deal of confusion has existed between the terms, synonyms, paronyms and antonyms, which describe Female Domination and its corollary: male submission. From our initial research, begun with the intent of bringing a little order to this lexical confusion, it became apparent, little by little, that the semantic nuances that we uncovered most often corresponded proportionally to the variations in Gynarchic social relationships, as they are lived, or in variations in the technique of male enslavement, or as actually practiced, or historically.

We thus wanted to pursue this line of inquiry, with the aim of establishing a taxonomy of all possible gynarchic systems, that might be lived collectively or individually, and of all the methods and stages leading to or bringing about these ideal social structures where only Women have power.

Unfortunately, even with limitless patience this task could never be carried out. How, indeed, could we imagine all possible situations in which a Woman dominates men? And how could we imagine all the possible methods She is likely to employ in order to reach her goals? It would be an insult even to describe a range within which she might operate, as one of the primary characteristics of Woman is precisely her brilliant imagination. But nonetheless we hope to have, if not a complete treatment of the subject, a treatment that exhausts the lexical possibilities given to Gynarchy by the dictionary.

Finally, it appears to be simpler, paradoxically, to begin our work with the goal we wish to reach (the enslavement of the male), and after having seen the various steps, arriving in the end at methods of enslavement and at several stages of training, and at the first encounter with the low creature who seems to us to be especially worthy of effort.

Would the above discussion encourage us to accept the validity of a formula, corresponding roughly to a male's social progression towards the gynarchic, and which would be stated:

(encounter + enslavement) + training = slavery.

But this would put on the same level a specific incident (the encounter), a state (slavery), the passage from one state into another (enslavement) and a process (training), and that is obviously not admissible within the framework of a semantically rigorous analysis.

It would be preferable instead to combine facts with facts and states with states, which could give rules of structural transformations of the type:

slavery = enslavement + training.

However it is appropriate, before formulating any rules, to set down the logical order of the transformations:

a) The progressive states of the male :

state Ø ± subjugation [86] ± submission ± slavery,

b) The descriptive names of the males :

inferior ± subordinate [87] ± submissive ± slave,

c) Of the corresponding titles of the Woman in charge :

Initiatrix ± Instructress [88] ± Dominatrix ± Mistress,

d) And of the stages which delineate training :

conditioning ± domestication ± enslavement.

Logical process that could be so figured :

FEMALE TITLE	Training Steps	Male positions	Male titles
INITIATRIX		state Ø	inferior
	conditioning		
INSTRUCTRESS		subordination	subordinate
	domestication		
DOMINATRIX		submission	submissive
	enslavement		
MISTRESS		slavery	slave

With our terminology in place, it is now possible for us to take up each term, or each degree of gynarchic progression again, feminine as well as masculine, and to create an analytical description that will allow us to formulate definitions of concepts, so that we may study our methods and observe the results.

Our study will not be chronological, beginning instead at the end of training, as if the cartesian male never mattered, but rather conversely and progressively, reached by average possibilities, the ideal of our realistic premises, in order to the necessity of each phase, and, above all, to move from the simplest to the most complex.

A - THE SLAVERY OF THE MALE, AT THE IDEAL, FINAL STAGE

The masculine ideal is naturally the factotum, etymologically expressed by, "*Do everything!*" What Woman has never dreamt of having at least one man to whom she could give a single order, beginning and ending with, "*Do everything!*" and after having pronounced it, never having to think about it again. Alas, "*factotum*" has too many positive connotations to be appropriate for a slave. Only the timid bourgeois women frightened by words will be satisfied. Gynarchy prefers the simple word slave, sometimes ennobled by the Latin synonym servus.

Let us note that Latin did not give Gynarchy only the terms *servus* and *factotum*. The Mistress, who has trained and posses a servus, will rarely be satisfied with only this servile exclusivity. She will soon need, in her *ergastulum* [89], a *famulus* to guard her, an *adstetrix* to keep, an *unctor* to maintain her fragrances, a *aplipilarus* to depilate, a *nutritor* for nourishment, a *trotactror* [90] to massage her, a *dropacistus* to clean her various natural openings, a *bajulus* to carry her, and a *cubicularus* to be used for service in bed.

And will return to the happy time of the *mancipium*, a male-object owned in totality and acquired through capture or purchase. The richest Women (or the most intrepid) will use a *supellex*, as a table or a living lamp. When Women take power, and we think that will be soon, we must be very precise with the names and labels which we will affix to our servants, and Latin, as we have seen, will be very useful.

B - THE ENSLAVEMENT OF THE MALE, AND HIS GRADUATION FROM STUDIES

As men formerly became Knights in a ceremony called dubbing, the male will obtain, under Gynarchy, the honor of receiving the title of "slave to a Woman" by the ceremony of Enslavement. After having been subordinate to an Instructress, then subjugated by a Dominatrix, the male will finally obtain the right to belong body and soul to a Mistress, to finally enter into slavery.

The Mistress will organize the ceremony as she pleases, if she considers it necessary. She might require a signed contract, but in practice will prefer an infibulation or an amputation symbolizing the male's enslavement, to plainly mark the irrevocability of his new masculine status.

If it was not done at the time of Domestication, the Mistress will indelibly affix her name or initial on the body of her slave, from now on her *mancipium*. The most durable marks are those made by a branding iron, which can be used to create aesthetically pleasing marks easily, even by a Woman who is somewhat awkward.

The Mistress will make the most of the Enslavement, if she wishes, by renaming her slave [91], and especially by assigning him new tasks or functions that are harder for him, and which will therefore bring more satisfaction to him, even if they are only temporary. One should not forget that the even as the Mistress makes a new acquisition, a new life that is intensely productive and enriching also begins for the male newly promoted into slavery.

C - THE TRAINING OF THE MALE, TRUE FEMININE PERFORMANCE

In our first diagram, between the state and slavery, the male moves through two distinct periods of training, subjugation and slavery. Between the two, there is a symbolic event and very important ritual: Domestication. The true gynarchic problem is situated exactly between subjugation and true submission, at the time of Domestication, the time when the male agrees to become a domestic, a servant.

It is easy, even for a young Mistress, to give a directive to a male and see the latter follow it without balking; it is more complex to give him an order (perhaps the same one) the execution of which intrinsically implies his inferiority and submission. Semantically, it is the difference between these sentences:

1) *This evening, darling, you will do the dishes !*

2) *Do the dishes quickly, darling !*

Even if each one of these sentences has the same practical result ("darling" does the dishes), the first implies a certain freedom of choice, in spite of the implicit order of the Instructress, while the second makes the authority of the Dominatrix explicit and does not leave an alternative to the subjugated.

These nuances make up the art of the female domination. And, to stay with the example of the dishes, marking his lost manhood, one can imagine a progression in the formulation of this order given by the Woman to the man:

a) *Do you want to do my dishes, my darling ?*

The Womyn recognizes that it is about HER dishes.

b) *Would you like to do the dishes for me, darling ?*

"For me" is ambiguous. Is it the ACTION of doing the dishes which is in place of the Womyn, or the man himself who must do it FOR her?

c) *Do the dishes quickly, darling !*

This is no longer a request, but an order.

d) *Do your dishes quickly, X...*

The possesive, implicating a specifical male duty, makes the imperative exclamation point unnecessary.

e) *The dishes, flunkey (or slave, etc.) !*

The "darling", via his new name, has finally found a functional appellation.

f) *Dishes !*

There is not more need for a handle, nominal, functional or diminutive. Soon, snapping the fingers will suffice...

But our present interest, in our study of the tactics of training, is the precise nature of the differences between sentences 1) and 2) or, in the second formulation, the orders b) and c). Between the two what we call, for convenience, the domestication of the male, has occurred. From a "service" that he provides, at the request of his Teacher, in b), the subjugated in the course of training passes, into c), where he has a duty to follow the Dominatrix's order.

If he does not comply with b), the male incurs neither reprimand nor quarrel. If he disobeys c), he is eligible for punishment(s) that may be more or less severe. It is the path between these two phrases, which requires a relative subtlety to understand and internalize, which in fact decides the success of the gynarchic home, and whether or not the male will slide into slavery.

This path must be gradual, progressing slowly, sometimes slipping backwards, and then restarting. The Instructress must sometimes employ the type b) formulation for her orders, other times the type c), and she must never become discouraged. Very soon, the Woman will feel the moment when she will be able to give orders in complete freedom, without carefully phrased remarks.

The male, previously conditioned for a few weeks or months, will be domesticated from now on.

When this stage is reached, the training must perfect itself, not only through learning, on the part of the male, of a obedience-reflex (natural coinciding with the establishment of an instinctive feminine authority in the beginning Dominatrix), but also by a consensual euphoria in the newly domesticated, taken from the punishments received for disobedience or for doing a poor job of carrying out female orders.

It is only at that time, after the graduation of tasks to be carried out in the service of the Dominatrix, and the punishments that are granted to him by her, that one can begin to see the enslavement of the applicant.

D - INITIAL STATE AND CONDITIONING

It is said that the first step is the most difficult. And this first step towards the gynarchic method is the most delicate and the most complex, for both the future slave and the future Mistress. It is necessary for the Woman to abandon her habits, jettison her taboos, and overcome her apprehensions.

At first, it is necessary for the Instructress to be quite conscious of her goal (the TOTAL enslavement of the male whom she has chosen), of the foreseeable difficulties (his probable resistance to enslavement), of the various efforts and the many sacrifices which she will have to put up with before succeeding in her task (wasted time, the repetition of training exercises, an environment that is sometimes difficult, etc.).

She should know that once the process has been set in motion, the Woman will no longer be able to be a follower, because if she does, she will have to withstand the sordid aggressive, and animalistic reaction the male always has when he regains his natural advantage.

So long as she constantly keeps her objective in mind, the Woman, slowly but surely, will succeed in her project. And she will have the ineluctable joy, not only of becoming a respected Instructress, but of seeing her slave submitting readily and slipping into the euphoria of slavery. But this training can be carried out satisfactorily only with the strict observance of a rigorous method, and a great deal of personal discipline.

We will summarize here, for the benefit of the novice Instructress, some of the fundamental rules and the methods which have been shown to be effective. For a more thorough understanding of the psychosexual techniques of gynarchic conversion, the Instructress should refer to the theoretical works quoted in our bibliography.

1) OMNIPRESENCE OF GYNARCHIC REFERENCES.

In your home, and all around you, it is necessary for there to be a maximum of objects d'art and works about Gynarchy (photographs, drawings or paintings representing of the Women dominating or killing men, novels depicting a world of Amazons or Gynarchists in action [93], video-cassettes inspired by the same themes, technical on the subject of Gynarchy, reviews of female domination or bulletins of Gynarchist organizations, etc.), and of objects which, in your environment, can imply, with regard to the male, your superiority or your cruelty (scientific books, warlike weapons, objects, instruments of torture, etc).

2) CONSTANT DOMINANT ATTITUDE.

Under no circumstances should a Woman follow – obey – an order emanating from a male, nor tolerate his giving one. Naturally, the opposite will become typical, and little by little, a rule.

Also, the Initiator will have to become accustomed to the dominant position. If both are sitting, the Woman must ALWAYS take the most comfortable seat, and/or highest. During a discussion, she must be seated while the man does address himself while standing. She must be on top during the sex act, etc.

3) USE OF MALE DESIRE.

It is the male, which desires the body of the Woman. She must thus enflame the desire of the male, satisfying it gradually, but only in exchange for progressive submission. From the first contact, the Woman must insist upon these exchanges. The least kiss, the least caress and, a fortiori, the least sexual contact must be granted only in the other hand of a manifest proof of submission (I will kiss you if you do the dishes, make love when you do the housework, sleep with you if you transfer your wages to my account, etc).

4) SPONTINAITY AND THE NECESSITY OF PUNISHMENT.

It can start with a tap on the cheek, by withholding dessert or sex, but little by little, the punishment of the male for bad behavior must become normal, legal, until he knows that he risks imprisonment, the whip, or torture in the event of pranks, of transgressions, or rebellion.

Gradually, the slap can become more severe, then a blow from the belt and, finally, the whip. Imperceptibly and gradually, the male must accept increasingly serious and physically painful corporal punishment.

5) GYNARCHIC THEORY

Little by little, the moral and physical superiority of the Instructress must become reveal itself to the male as self-evident, and as an irresistible force. For that, in addition to the intellectual justification the subordinate needs to justify his penchant for servitude, the Woman must chip away at him with expressions, slogans, precepts, proverbs, sayings that help his memory, which the male will adopt as life rules to which he can always refer to know how to act. Some examples:

- *Every husband must show submission to his wife*
- *Beaten by his Wife, happy at heart.*
- *What Women want, God wants.*
- *A Girl's wishes are never faults.*
- ...

6) CONTRACTUALISATION.

Very soon, it will be necessary to present rules, formulated orally at first, then written, establishing in a progressive but indissoluble way the Woman's rights and the duties of the male. We propose, in order to give a name to this first step towards Gynarchy, to call this contract governing elaborating gynarchic relations, signed and respected, Conditioning.

Finally, having presented in reverse order the various stages and the various periods of gynarchic life, we have, while defining, named (or christened) each one of them. This was not only an end but a means as well, allowing us, among other things, to conceptualize the control of the male, and bring about, consequently, the rapid ascent of Gynarchy.

FOURTH PART : A BETTER WORLD FOR WOMEN IN FULL BLOOM
and disciplined men

I - THE POLITICAL TAKEOVER

1. Male psycho-intellectual regression and its socio-cultural consequences.

The 20th century was marked, in particular in its first two thirds, by an intensification of the struggles of Feminist, its two world wars, mainly intended to suppress them under the virile ones and fallacious patriotic pretexts, that could not be right. With this latent and increasingly precise threat that an emancipated and conquering Femininity made on its usurped powers, the male reacted by the creation of conditioning media, like television, the multiplication of debilitating pseudo-philosophical theories and the resurgence of religious fanaticism.

But these frightened and criminal chauvinist decision makers, forgot one vital thing, their self protection. And, as Womyn, unconsciously, rationally or thanks to their sixth dense, were more or less prepared for this unhealthy and petty reaction, the principal victims of this desperate counter-offensive are to be precisely the male elements of these sacrificed generations. When one uses as a last weapon the propagation of illiteracy, intolerance, ignorance and stupidity,

it is well to expect that the first contaminated, as with most of the other epidemics, are the males. And it is that of which we are well obliged to report today.[94]

Just like the young boy at school, the adult male at this inhuman end of the century became limited, malicious, uncultivated and is tragically in a manifest position of inferiority, or even of total dependence, with respect to the Womyn. He even understands with great difficulty that his psycho-intellectual state, near to the abject, is only the result of an intrinsic fault which he cultivated instead of circumscribing and proscribing it by subjecting, without condition, hesitation nor regret, to his partner, either a Lady, a Womyn, a Grrl or a young Grrl who is by nature superior psychologically and intellectually compared to him.

This stammering awakening, that with a little understanding we all can note in our unfortunate companions, alas has thus deteriorated so much due to his male ego that only a servitude, total or partial, can dissolve it effectively. One cannot sweep away millennia of male chauvinist certainty in a few years of Female predominance. However, little by little, the male admits his inferiority and accepts a certain social regression to the Womyn's profit. Indications do not lack (higher rates on automobile insurance for the young male drivers, the teaching profession almost entirely Feminized, Female decision makers on almost all the levels of the administration, Justice, etc.) that the total social tendency is with the Female preponderance in all fields (policy, commercial, convivial, etc).

The evidence, and if the few males which still obstinately refuse their defeat do not irreversible cause a third world war, the twenty first century will see the result of this evolution and its outcome, with the profit of this long fight for power to the Womyn. The problem of unemployment will pragmatically be solved by the only reasonably desirable reforms, the confiscation by the Womyn of all the decision-making jobs and the more or less general assignment of the males to manual and servile work.

But we will have to take care not to fall into the same traps that the males did when they themselves had absolute power. It will be necessary, of course, to separate them from all the functions of responsibility but however to keep some of them, among the most submissive and adapted to Female supremacy, in apparent situations of decision making to show their fellows who would find hard to swallow their dependence but which, fortunately, will remain always also easy to fool. In the family, one will naturally need to confine them to the domestic tasks but nevertheless to sometimes agree to direct them, at least verbally, in certain fields manifestly more delicate as the kitchen, for example, and the decoration of the house. In the same way, if the total sexual freedom of the Womyn and polyandry must be universally institutionalized and not cause any dispute it will have despite everything to tolerate, for example in the form of loan with another Womyn or under pretext of erotic formation in a specialist, a certain infidelity of her husbands, thus giving the illusion of a certain reciprocity. All this comes within the province of common sense and will not pose any problem in the newborn Gynarchy. But still it is necessary that each Womyn knows which male reactions to be expecting from now on for the few years or the few decades which separate us from final success and by which control to answer them. A good theoretical knowledge of etiology and semiology, of the current psycho-intellectual regression of the male will give the Womyn called to guide the advent Gynarchist the theoretical bases necessary to the use of these same male intrinsic flaws to the profit of the ideal society in construction.

The debilitating psychological degeneration that the males of the human species undergo today, just like their manifest progressive stupidity, must obviously become the Female weapons for the radical social change in preparation. The intrinsically male tendency to unload responsibilities, which one notes in the politicians as in the simple fathers of families, (the former discharge on technicians, and still some technicians, of all the incomprehensible technical problems for them, the latter give up to their more qualified partners the financial, functional direction and morals of their family which they cannot assume), will be the key to Womyn being able acquire power.

When, on all the decision making levels of society, the global to the family unit, the male, as he already is doing gradually, will have the absolute obligation to refer about it to one of the Womyn , there will be required nothing more than one small blow to give so that the declining male chauvinist world rocks definitively and irrevocably to nothing.

2. Revolution or reform?

Gynarchic theory, primarily revolutionary since it aims at a radical upheaval of the practices and systems of thought, however admits that its advent can be done without violence, via certain reforms relatively not very constraining, like those aiming at the fields of Health, Contraception, the Retirement.[95]

a) Health in the Gynarchic system.

The system of health care of the modern world that we desire will have to comprise about same medical specialization's as today. However, it is the management of medicine known as general practitioner, of current consumption, which is entirely to be re-examined. The problems of health which do not belong to the specialized fields cannot be tackled and dealt with in a satisfactory way by experts not having a global vision of the anatomy, physiology and psychology of Womyn. This is why, so that a general practitioner is effective and does not have unceasingly to return patients to specialists, it is necessary that an internist has sufficient

specialized training in Gynecology. The future of mass consumer medicine necessarily progresses by a Gynecological approach to the current problems of health. The Womyn will thus benefit therefore from both a global and at the same time personalized solution their problems of health and will be treated finally as women.

In addition, one can note that the veterinary who in medicine, is exceptionally qualified in all the fields, suffers from an arbitrary limitation of its field of activities. Indeed, the Veterinary

surgeons of today who make true miracles as regards animal care would gain considerably in practical knowledge and effectiveness if they could in parallel deal with certain small medical and/or surgical problems of humans. Indeed, it is not terribly pejorative, for a doctor able to operate a gorilla or a dog in open heart and to cure raging fevers, not to have the right to make a diagnosis and prescribe an ordinary aspirin or tranquilizer for a human which would need some? Obviously, the Veterinary surgeons could happily undertake the care of the population

unconcerned by, on the one hand, the general Gynecology of which we come to show the need and, on the other hand, the medical fields specialized like Podiatry.

Thus, we could delineate three great families of experts: Specialists (orthopedists, podiatrists, etc), the Gynecologists general practitioners for Womyn and Veterinary surgeons for the animals and human males. The dichotomy, specialized medicine and general practitioner which does not correspond any more to contemporary medical reality will be happily supplanted by the triple functional distinction: medicine of specialties for the complex problems of health, general and Gynecology for the specifically Female problems and veterinary medicine with its widened field of competence, in particular including the medical and surgical problems of human males and the specific problems of this last (venerology, repressive castration or with the contraceptive goal, humane or repressive euthanasia, etc).

These improvements of our system of health would also have as a consequence, in addition to much better medical results, in particular for the Womyn, a considerable improvement of the budget of Social Security since, on the one hand, the Womyn would not any more, in general and except in complex cases be asking for the intervention of a specialist, that to consult only one doctor (if not a general practitioner then a gynecologist, as it is alas still the case currently) and the males could reasonably hope to find in the Veterinary surgeon a response to 99 % of their health problems.

b) Contraception in Gynarchy.

In spite of all of the progress of modern science, castration remains the most effective means of contraception and the cheapest. It is indisputable. However, this contraceptive method, because undoubtedly of its final nature and some other minor disadvantages, remains rather little used currently, especially, of course, in the patriarchal societies which still remain, in particular in Africa. Gynarchy will take care to rehabilitate and give to bring back in style this healthy and effective practice.

Certain Womyn will obviously not find it beneficial to castrate their male companions or servants: it is those which know sexual pleasure only vaginal and or which cannot be satisfied with phallic substitutes to obtain the orgasm. Admittedly, it is an obvious deficiency of knowledge as regards Female sexuality (even of a regrettable lack of sexual practices with Female instruments and or of same sex partners) but one will not be able to condemn those which, not wishing to have children, will not require this sacrifice of their male partner to preserve the use of the same bodies which to them bring pleasure. To prefer castration with the condom, for the pill (or the moyenâgeux vaginal contraceptives), it is physically necessary to be a psychologically a free Woman and, conscious of mediocrity of the pleasure obtained using the male and aware of the enormous progress made in the field of Female pleasure by erotic gadgets

and chemical aphrodisiacs. Moreover, in Gynarchy, the male, even castrated, can very easily be conditioned with the regular execution of erotic handling, to possibly doubled oral operations, which will be able him to satisfy their partner fully, in particular if these last are primarily clitoral orgasms.

The Womyn eager not to have a child (or more children), that by fear of the labor pains, preference for the adoption or predilection for extra-uterine fertilization with selected sperm, will have to choose between the two sound techniques of castration of Her males :

1) the ablation of only the testicles (if the Wife or the partner of the male is heterosexual and or in the case referred to above).

2) the complete ablation of the genital apparatus of the male (if his Wife or partner is Lesbian exclusive or unfortunately frigid).

N.B. As for the bisexual Womyn, She will have to specify Her preferences at the time when they will fill the official request of castration of their companion (and in any event at least an hour before the operation).

Castration undoubtedly fell in disuse because of all the chauvinist taboos surrounding the Female's pleasure (saphism condemned or reserved for the magazines and films " for men ", and vibrators sold in specialized shops surrounded with an air of shame, aphrodisiacs reserved to the men and for limited circulation, etc...).

Thus, by giving again a rise to this extraordinarily effective contraceptive method, Gynarchie will contribute, on the one hand, to a significant increase in the comfort of Womyn (no possibility of "accident " , no more expensive I.V.G., or tiresome daily doses of pills, etc.) and, in addition, through the Goddess, of chemical and the erotic gadgets, with a very beneficial revitalization of Female eroticism, as the driving principle of the world of tomorrow.

3. Other secondary measurements.

a) Suppression of the administrative formalities concerning males.

All this monstrous and expensive management of State-Civil (death, birth notification, marriage, etc.) is not needed, at least with regard to the males. A simple declaration (in a space reserved on the forms of annual income tax return, for example) by each Womyn, having, having given birth or having buried one or more males, would be enough each year, in particular for the statistics. Many Female jobs as Secretary of Town hall etc. would be thus simplified and would thus become more attractive.

b) Reduced schooling of the males.

The problem of Teaching is crucial. The generalized creation of I.M.E.G.[96] is of course desirable but immediate measurements are essential. It is not useful, for example, to teach Arts and the Literature to a male, whose only function, at the end of its studies, will be to be the servant of a

Womyn and or to do manual work for Her. What purpose is served by teaching a foreign Language to a male which in the last analysis, will have to understand only some orders whose translation would largely be on sheet of paper (upright!, slept!, here!, outside!, lick!, drink!, eat!, etc.) After (or during) the psychological training of our poor miserable inferior companion, it would be enough to give them two or three years of training as apprenticeship in the tasks which will be required of him (in particular in the domestic sciences and the care of the Female body), together with a few elementary concepts of Gynarchic Morals and Philosophy, to make a

completely acceptable and functional male of him. True scientific and cultural teaching, reserved to the Grrls, would become really effective, appealing and attractive. The trades of Education,

already almost completely Feminized, would then become less painful and attractive, which would bring without any doubt many young Womyn to want to practice them.

c) Right of non-assistance to male in danger or suffering.

A simple refusal of the Receptionist to accept, to the Hospital or the Private clinic, males not-accompanied by their Mother, Sister, Concubine, Tutor or Mistress, would reduce considerably the task of the Nurses and their assistants and would also have as a result a new passion for this Female employment. This measure, in time, could be extended to the Old people's home. However, it would be inhuman and not very hygienic to refuse to the male the right to a Crematorium.

d) Exemption for the justifications for male euthanasia.

To put an end to the life of a male, with an obviously charitable or hygienic aim, should not be any more an act subjected to preliminary authorization or later justification of the Womyn decision-maker. The administrative, legal and legal formalities which block today the execution of this act of pity and or elementary social hygiene make it almost unrealizable by the one making this decision, even in all full knowledge of the cause. Many feel obliged to put an end illegally to the days of their unhappy companion, which is unacceptable and obliges sometimes the Womyn to use ingeniousness methods to achieve Her ends without fearing administrative annoyances. A simple declaration on the honor, written hand of the Mother, Sister, Concubine, Tutor or Mistress, indicating, in conscience, the date and the reasons of Her decision should be amply sufficient to justify morally and administratively this courageous act. We would very quickly be relieved of all these males in a bad physical or mental, which encumber us and, in

addition, the stations which would be thus released could be reserved to the Womyn precisely and, naturally, in first place that would have practiced the act of creative euthanasia.

II - FOR AN EXCLUSIVELY FEMALE MANAGEMENT OF MILITARY, POLICE AND PENITENTIARIES

That the men are the only ones to go to the front in time of war while the Womyn continue to enjoy life, without them or with those which remain, is an elementary civic and social principle

that no one thinks of calling into question. However, it is probable that our valiant soldiers would be much more effective if they were subordinates exclusively to officers and noncommissioned officers of the Female sex, at the time of ground operations or during their time of obligatory active service. Several elements show us the undeniable advantages which will result from a real Female Supremacy in the military body.

1 - National service.

Initially, psychologically, the teenager called up for military service will much more easily submit to a Female authority which carries out a continuity between the maternal authority, whose child sees himself deprived for this period, and the absolute power under whose authority he will soon be of his Mistress when being given to Her in marriage. To pass from the supervision of the Mother to that of the Wife by the intermediary of a pseudo-virile authority is one of these aberrations to which men are accustomed in the sectors where they still prevail. Undoubtedly it is

because of this stupidity that so many couples are seen today to be torn by divorce[97], the man temporarily having lost the values of the Female Authority and thinking his manhood dishonored by being subject to a Womyn again.

With the military service, four types of lesson are taught and each one of them needs to be inculcated in the young recruits by Womyn-officers.

a) Handling of the weapons.

The Womyn, because of their greater overall intelligence and their natural tact, are more able to understand, and thus to teach, delicate handling which the mechanisms of the weapons require to use.

On the other hand the attraction of deadly weapons which are perfectly usable even by very Grrls, by that time well more useful to them.

b) Physical Training.

A woman, knows better than anyone which are the tasks that She must assign to Her companions, weather they are assigned to him as voluntary slaves, servants, lovers or a simple

husband, and to what training he must subject for a good result.

Ultimately and obviously, the physical condition of the men (which, is determined only for their being better able to serve their intellectually privileged partners) is the business of the Womyn to decide and it is quite natural that these last direct with an iron hand the various obligatory body exercises their subordinates.

c) The Assignment and Supervision of the chores.

As Mistress of the house (or future Mistress if it is about a young Grrl), the Womyn non-commissioned officer who will see Herself in charge of the distribution and the supervision of the chores will teach to the soldiers all the unwelcome tasks [98] or services which await them from the very start of their married life or their entry into the service of a Mistress. Of course, the higher ranking of each young conscript will think of the future wellbeing of all the young Womyn who will collect the fruits of Her necessary severity.

d) The training of docility.

The military service is the privileged moment where the young person called " becomes a man ", based upon the devotion he expresses.

That means the moment when he learns really and concretely to obey. The Womyn are obviously concerned most of all that the basic male training is accomplished as best as possible. For, of course, it is they who will derive later the advantages of the good training of their companions of the lower sex. It is thus good for them to supervise

conscientiously and to direct with firmness this second male education. The Womyn officers, in particular, will not forget to use the various punishments which the army places at their disposal to subdue the strong heads, knowing that inflicted punishments intelligently, even sometimes wrongfully, largely helps to forge the disciplined and flexible characters which they will like to see thereafter.

2 - The role of the Womyn officers in time of war.

War, if there must be war, can be well carried out only by Womyn. She only can advisedly and judge opportunity of the sacrifice of such or such soldier. Since it is Her which gives him life, She only must be entitled morally to decide destiny of the man of which She is the natural mission is to be sacrificed for Her.

It is obvious that a Womyn officer sending a soldier to death will have weighed wisely for and against it and will have humanly measured the consequence of Her

decision, more especially as a Womyn knows better than anyone what valid service well trained men can do.

Lastly, it is in the nature of the man to sacrifice himself for the Womyn and She by giving a dangerous order, even by explicitly sending a man to death, has much more chances than a male soldier of being obeyed without protest.

3 - Police and prisons.

In certain states of the USA, it has been several years that with success one readily finds entrusted to Women the guard of male prisoners, including those in maximum security. In a recent report on the

American prisons, one could hear the testimony of several Supervisors of Penitentiaries. If a Guardian confesses to exert Her authority on the male delinquents with a joy which often its prisoners share, another admits misusing sometimes its capacity on the hardest of the prisoners of the prison and experiencing an unquestionable pleasure with these abuses. In the quarters of the condemned to death, Female comings and goings, even punctuated sometimes by some brutalities necessary towards most recalcitrant, are a relief for those which, following unforgivable actions, must finish very soon with the life. A Female smile, even ironic, always brings a little softness to the last minutes of the condemned.

The police force also gains much with progressive feminization in progress. The Womyn, more understanding, have much better relationship with the civil population. As for the delinquents, more or less always in search of a Maternal reprimand, they much less easily yield to the injunctions of a male police officer than those of the Female police officers that they meet now, which allows these last also to appear to be more firm and, consequently, much more effective.

Increasingly, the authorities in power choose Women to run their armies, police and prisons. Almost all the so-called Western world from now on will be subjected, at one time or another, during their national service, to the authority of their Females just as are the delinquents and prisoners. The majority of these young Women volunteers, because of their natural superiority, are almost all incorporated in the ranks or higher levels of the military, police or administrative hierarchy. For now the young people called and many of the delinquents have relatively little to do with the higher sex and must generally undergo the sad misused authority of machos.

But fortunately, the young recruit; the prisoner or the criminal sometimes crosses the path of these Women of authority who also procures him his uniform and his rank. Then, timidly, the young soldier, like the prisoner assumes the rightful position of respect and puts himself at attention and finds himself in seventh heaven when She returns his salute while sometimes giving him a condescending smile.

III - GYNARCHY AND FULL EMPLOYMENT

1 - The Man.S.O.U.M.

a) A help for the young unmarried Womyn activates

Mainly, the European voters are favorable to drastic governmental measures in favor of full employment and against the waste of unemployment allowances. The Gynarchists also favor this. In particular, "Gynarchy International" proposed the idea of Man.S.O.U.M. (MANdatory Service Of Unemployed Males) which benefits from a very strong wave of sympathy, as much on behalf of the taxpayers whose taxes are used for the compensation for the unemployed person as for working Womyn , first recipients of this future measure.

Let's recall that it will act, everywhere in the world, to compel the male bachelor, claimants of employment, in return for the allowances that they receive from the state, one obligatory work period, of thirty hours per week more or less, that they should do at the domicile and under the authority of an, unmarried and working Womyn. These services can be of any kind, including merely domestic, will offer the immense advantage of avoiding the sometimes dangerous idleness of the young unemployed person while at the same time promoting the independence and the work of Women.

b) A solution to the divorce of the unemployed person

Of course, in spite of the excellent foundations of this future law, it will probably be difficult to avoid some abuses. Some local Directors of the agency for employment won't fail to use their legal powers, not only to take advantage personally of services of the best male Claimants, which is relatively natural and will carry hardly any consequence, but also to PUNISH most of the unemployed divorced persons whose management of the allowances and the obligatory work will fall to them.

In fact, it is likely that some leaders of this organization, confirmed or converted Gynarchists , will have the pleasure of assigning to any divorced Womyn Her ex-husband (if, of course, he benefits from an unemployment allowance) so that he carries out all domestic or other work his ex-Wife will ask him to do.

These new relations between the subordinate ex-husband to an ex-Wife become his manager will doubtless have very positive results. Some Womyn will take advantage of their new authority to re-conquer a flighty husband and others, more calculating, to institute such a report of strengths in their favor that the unemployed person will nearly see himself obligated to submitting for life to Her use, for their greater mutual satisfaction. Other Womyn again, more perfectionist, will want the services of their ex - husband in the squalid goal to take vengeance for a messy divorce.

Thus, thanks to the Man.SO.U.M., many, meeting in part to transform their ex - husband legally into a servant, probably won't be content with that and will proceed day after day to a psychological and systematic destruction of the weak and intrinsically lower being that the law will have put back into their hands.

A lot of these males will become stooges in the hands of a Womyn married by chance and deceived accidentally. He will become presumably Her slave and will accept quickly, after a minimum Gynarchist conditioning, to remain permanent in the domicile of his new manager, and without limitation of the work time.

Putting completely to use their social and psychological superiority on their ex-husbands, the divorced Womyn will be able to easily and legally collect, in their own bank account the totality of the allowances of unemployment of their docile servant.

And if former friends of the new servant try, with the amused authorization of his manager, to argue the newly submitted male, he will thanks to the virtues of an efficient Gynarchic psychological treatment, will confess to them to be fully conscious of the wrong that he done to his ex - Wife while divorcing and is very anxious to make amends to her. Finally, very satisfied with his fate, treated fairly and without excessive severity by his ex - Wife sound, he will finally discover himself at his true place while remaining in her personal service.

As for the jobless person's new Female employer, She will only be shown to be delighted by Her servant and their new relationship, much more in conformity to their reciprocal temperaments than a superficial and sterile union.

The directors of the ANPE will be just as delighted with this turn of the events and will certainly feel like fairies giving back life to divided couples.

c) Toward the full employment of the males

Thus, very quickly, even while making abstraction of the special and particularly profitable case of the unemployed divorced person, the male bachelors, in particular the young, will be formed then probably without problems by their young managers recycled in jobs of service, if, however (and as likely in the major part of the cases), they don't prefer to keep their allowances and work as the personal servant of a young Womyn to whom they will be able to contribute to the personal success of or, at least, to the comfort and to the well-being of that She naturally deserves.

Thus, as soon as they reach the official age of entry into the active life, all young males will be very quickly and totality assigned to the tasks that are appropriate to them. Those that would not find place on the farms or in the factories of production, of transportation and maintenance, will see themselves, on the one hand, duly salaried and, on the other hand, usefully assigned to the service of some young Womyn, in a setting of industry or administration, in activity in the handicraft trade or a liberal profession.

2 - male Farms.

Modern technology, still badly exploited, again because of the few male decision makers still in place, will allow the reigning Gynocracy to proceed very easily to big concentrations of the male population. Indeed, the technique, now perfected to the point, of the electro - cerebral implant, makes completely possible the surveillance of several hundreds of male workers by a small team of a dozen Supervisors sufficiently equipped.

Initially a numeric microphone - transmitter will be implanted, safely, in the brain of every male to be supervised electronically. This electronic implant, equipped with a personalized code, will be locatable by parabolic type radar at a distance of several score of kilometers.

On each of the monitors [99] reproducing the radar - picture, the Supervisors will have a precise view of the geographical situation of every micro - emitter therefore, of every male, and, thanks to the codes displayed on their screens, of the identity of each of the male subjects at each site.

It is therefore unnecessary to put in peril the remainder of the Gynarchic society and to be able to proceed to big concentrations of males, in particular in farming zone where it is made necessary in the setting of an extensive agricultural, and ecological production of quality. One will be able to isolate thus in vast Farms, like the soviet kolkhoz example, the farm workers selected by the professional advisors, the recalcitrant males in the Gynarchy and give them justice.

The computer of the male Farm will replace the close supervision of the guards which will be advantageous and less dangerous for them.

Messages of digital orders [100] will be distributed to the males all along their day of labor through the intermediary of loudspeakers situated on all the extent of the Farm. Their displacements will be permanently visible on the monitor and recorded daily. The control of work done will everywhere possible be by circuit video (in the barns and the shops) and by direct verification of the Supervisors (after, of course, the return of the males to their stalls) where the control of video is difficult, in the fields in particular.

With Her computer, a qualified Supervisor should be able to direct about a thousand males, sometimes sending them to such or such field, then bringing back them toward the collective showers, the dining hall or the dormitories. In the same way, equipped with the sophisticated weapons required for their profession and having a special vehicle or a small helicopter well equipped, one or two other Supervisors only will be in charge of suppression of males who commit infringements of the regulations or to deal with males who are too lazy. Finally, one or two supplementary Womyn should be sufficient to manage the daily life of the male workers of the Farm, the ordering and distribution of food, sanitary conditions, withdrawal or elimination of any disruptive elements, etc. On the whole therefore, considering the maximum period of the Feminine work recommended by the Gynarchists [101] (three times six hours weekly), two or three teams of twelve Supervisors would be amply sufficient to direct a Farm of a thousand of heads [102].

Obviously, on our Farms, to avoid the depression of the males, due to continuous quasi – absence of Females, and to elevate in the same way the masculine aggressiveness that can be only moderated by Womyn, the cohort of workers should live in a medium of an exclusively Female material environment and to be plunged permanently in an omnipresent ambient Femininity. The voices of the loudspeakers, as we saw, will be naturally Feminine and suggestive, but also the decoration of the stalls and the various other places of life of the males should be carried out solely with portraits of Womyn, of the illustrations Gynarchists, and of graphics enhancing the reigning Femininity.

The distractions (essentially audiovisual) of the males should be centered completely on the Womyn: studies on the psychology or the sexuality of the Feminine gender [103], documentaries on the daily life of the Womyn in the Gynarchist system, biographies of famous or anonymous Womyn, movies emphasizing the Feminine realities of the day, the progression of the standard of living of Womyn, etc.

Thus, peacefully and without excessive public expenses, and without having to mobilize too much good Feminine effort, the degenerate, recalcitrant males will be able to work usefully towards the comfort of their superior companions and to their supply of good food, while contributing efficiently to the suppression of unemployment.

3. The Feminine week of 3 days.

Rather than drown in endless controversy on a reduction of the amount of weekly work hours, some asserting the impossibility of this reform and others opting for a work week of 39, 37, perhaps of 35 hours, Gynarchist political thought brings new proposals and solutions whose logic has to bring to agreement all reactionary politicians and the pseudo revolutionaries.

The reduction of the time of work must obviously and rightfully benefit in the first place the fraction of population that has the most need and that will be better able to use this supplementary free time, that is obviously, to Womyn. Because they have the responsibility of the education of children, because society owes them social and political pre-eminence, Womyn are the most able to profit intelligently and fruitfully from the two weekly days diminution of work time.

Because it would be impossible to decrease the schedule of worked hours for all without harming the necessary productivity of the country and considering multiple viewpoints that confront us in this affair, it is necessary to create new jobs by this reduction of the duration of work of some. The solution is to create two types of work week: one reserved to males and narrowly framed having to be oriented towards productivity and output, the other, reserved to Womyn and liberated to the maximum of social and professional constraints, centred on education, culture and leisure.

The Gynarchy proposes therefore, in a first intermediate time, to combine a "male" work week of five full days with a "Feminine" work week of three days modifiable. The free time thus granted to Womyn will allow, them the substantial time of leisure for the benefit of their children, public businesses and their personal blooming, and also to create a massive program of the hiring of long unemployed males and youths.

Of course, local problems are likely to arise from the official institution of a Feminine week of 3 days. It will be necessary without doubt to envisage a temporary compensation system that will allow enterprises or administrators to push the male week to 6 or 6.5 days of work, a measure that would be, of course, only temporary.

But, during this period of unavoidable adaptation unemployment will disappear. All the inactive will ultimately find work presenting itself. Womyn will be able to profit from the free time thus released to them to improve not only their comfort, but also their family's in whose environment they socially and professionally grow and evolve.

Thus it is seen, with these few simple and efficient measures (to which one will add those, higher views, concerning the Teaching and the right to the euthanasia of males[104]), the Gynarchy will solve most human and social problems, including the most crucial of one our time, that sometimes makes the life of Womyn impossible to begin with, this real leprosy of unemployment.

IV - GYNARCHY AND SPIRITUALITY WOMYN' S DEIFICATION & MALE' S THINGIFICATION

1) The male slave : animal, vegetable or mineral ?

The dominant Women, owners of one or more slaves, often have a too summary vision of the psychology of the males which serve them. They have tendency (but it is a very normal reaction as soon as one starts to take the practice of the submission of the males) to compare their slave to an object, with a domestic robot stripped of feelings or psychology. It is a scientific error [105]. Admittedly, subjected male have a very rudimentary psychology which compares it more with an animal than with a human being. One educates him as an ass with carrot and the stick, other trains him like the rider trains up her circus horse, other still makes he acts by conditioned reflex like the dogs of Pavlov... This is perfectly exact. However its system of thought deserves all the same some analysis, therefore short and brief is it. The submissive has to interiorize his Mistress's tastes and ideas while he tries at the maximum to approach it by permanent imagination, and in real time, of her feelings of superior Woman of which he naturally cannot get the least idea. This psycho-sensory improvement beyond to which the submale has to be permanently compelled to go towards the female ideal (to which he cannot of course step claim) can also be transcended in a progressive cognitive renouncement.

His hybrid state, semi-human semi-animal, is often uncomfortable for the slave. His spirit always tended towards the unknown feelings and out of its attack which test the superior Women, and his Mistress in particular, work which it daily carries out for her and the worship that it dedicates to him in silence, undoubtedly helps him to live his natural

94

inferiority and his servile destiny but, alas, cannot be enough to make him forget him deep generic uselessness. It is for that that, often under the impulse of a a little psychological Mistress but sometimes by some personal impulse, engages the slave into a true process of reification which is very far from being detrimental, as well for him even as a fortiori for his Mistress.

There are, seems to us it, three great steps in this interesting "thingification" of the male.

a) The first is, to a certain extent, a "wall-step". The submale enters a house or an apartment to which it will be rivetted (with the illustrated direction, but also often with the literal meaning). He belongs to the residence of his Mistress as much as to herself. His horizon of life (which became by primarily domestic nature) is limited by the walls of her house and one of the principal tasks that he has to perform is to take care of the cleanliness and the arrangement of all that is locked up between these walls. His first identification with real space in which he is located, sometimes to which he is definitively connected [106], is a first step in the process of reification of subjected male.

b) The second stage is a "movable-step". The male attached to a place, and whose principal function is to take care of the maintenance of this one and what it contains, sometimes because in the way of which it is maltreated or simply been unaware of by the female population that it must be useful or, very often as, thanks to an acute and intrinsic conscience of his natural inferiority, feels obscurely as it is from a utilitarian point of view and psychologically much nearer to the pieces of furniture of the house than of the Women, far too superior to him, who live there regularly. Moreover, he accepts very easily (even appreciates from the first days of his enslavment !) to be used lengthily like any of the other pieces of furniture of his Mistress (stool, standard lamp, table, davit, etc, the movable possibilities of a male are innumerable...) [107].These other pieces of furniture, which are ultimately his principal companions, can become also its rivals. A subjected good used as footrest by a Woman will have in heart to remain at least as stable as a vulgar wood stool. He would be upset to see his Mistress preferring his vegetable made companion than himself ! Conversely, he will be proud of being able, contrary to his fellow-member coat rack, to advance until that which will have suspended, for example, her rainwears and her cap with its tended arms or on his head. Little by little, this movable function of the male must take the step on all its other more animal functions until, for example, not believe more that he is a slave washing the linen of his Mistress but indeed a washing machine improved in the course of use by this one or another Woman knowing to make it function.

c) Third is assimilation to the thing. Lastly, his fetishism helping him, the slave is often put to envy or be jealous of the clothing or the underclothing of his Mistress, especially when this one prohibits to him any direct contact with its divine body of Woman. During the washing with the hand of a support-throat or breeches, or during the meticulous sharpening of a dress, the submale will imagine this pretty linen stuck to the skin of its Mistress, unceasingly coming very close to her body and her forms, impregnating itself with her perfume and her intimate odor, all prohibited pleasures for him. Then he will appreciate very much more the choice a Woman can make to choose a wall cupboard like adequate place for putting up her slave. Higher stages of this wall cupboard being reserved to his Mistress' clothing, underclothing or shoes, the lowerstage affected to the male during his periods of rest or when his presence is undesirable in the residential parts of the Women. Slowly but ineluctably, the submale objectivises himself and becomes a useful thing. The process of reification is accomplished.

A " thinking " object, certainly, but object all the same, the male very quickly gains with being " thingified", and being compared to the remainder of her Mistress' trousseau. Here everything gains in clearness with these Womyn/male (or Mistres/slave, which returns to same) relations. A place for each thing and each thing in its place, known as popular wisdom. The dominant Woman will choose to penetrate this maxim in what is used as brain by his slave, while making him well understand that it indeed became really a thing, her thing, and that it must remain definitively in his place of thing, to let live the Women in their place of Women.

2) Another process for male reification : ON/OFF and STANDBY controls for slaves

In order to live in harmony with her slave, it is of utmost importance for a Mistress to invent and impose a code, sometimes a practical ritual, enablig her to put her submissive out of service when she does not need him or, more simply, whenever his presence or his activity bother her. With most her electric or electronic household appliances, a Woman usually has at her disposal a couple of controls, switches or push-buttons, generally identified with the words ON/OFF or I/O.

This is not the case, alas, with her natural slave, man. When our Mother Nature created the male to attend the needs of his superior companion, she did not decide to equip him with such mechanisms, for instance on his forehead or at the back of his head. Women must hence create by themselves special devices to provoke similar or identical results with their human servants.

It is certainly possible for a Mistress to have the representation of an electrical switch tattooed on her slave's forehead or cheekbone. The drawing can bear the ON/OFF inscription or any other clear terminology. The male is then instructed to perform immediately certain deeds, whenever a Woman's finger tip touches this part of his body (for instance : going into his kennel, his cupboard, or whatever location he has been assigned to, positioning himself there according to his Mistress's previously given commands, and stay motionless and quiet until a feminine finger touches the same spot again). Women who do not like complications will find an advantage to this method : ON/OFF procedures are identical for all the appliances used. In addition, it accelerates the reification process, it reinforces the submissive's status as a thing, and it persuades him even more, if possible, that he is by nature an owned object.

However some Women, for aesthetical reasons or because they fear negative comments, do not resort to such branding or tattooing. They use an oral code (connection/disconnection, for instance, or slave-on/ slave-off) which, when received by the slave's so-called brain, through his auditory canal, produces a similar effect. This saves the cost of tattooing, and avoids the small aesthetical damage. However, it has the inconvenient of forcing the Mistress to adress constantly her slave, a process which often induces him to forget that his status with respect to Women is only that of an object.

We will not comment on the following decision, which may be a bit extreme and is in any case of difficult implementation, by a Lesbian Mistress who wanted to deprive her slave of any human caracteristics. She had his torso tattooed with sensory controls corresponding to each of the domestic functions she had assigned him. During the first days, the slave needed to look at which spot was touched by his Mistress's forefinger in order to know what she expected from him. However, his inital errors were systematically punished and, quickly, pavlovian-type, unconsciously validated, reflexes replaced these few seconds of reflection. Since then, whenever a feminine forefinger touches one of these controls drawn on his torso, the slave immediately sets himslef to the task expected from him. It is not unreasonable to think that soon, with some over-talented or memory-gifted males, all Women will be able to program their slaves, even for several days ! It will look like a dream to all modern Mistresses who want to improve their comfort that such techno-psychological progress only requires, to be made possible, a little bit of imagination and know-how.

Besides the on/off control for her slave(s), a dominant Woman must definitely plan to have a STANDBY control. Indeed, she may need to be able to disactivate a male temporarily, for a short period, without having to send him to his assigned location, often difficult to access and remote from where his Mistress(es) live. The slave's standby control (or the sensor tattooed on his body) must correspond to a single position (in general kneeling with head bowed down), with total lack of motion and absolute silence. The slave should not have to move away to take this position. The control is extremely handful when receiving a phonecall, an unexpected visitor, and in thousands of other situations.

A Woman who masters those two passive functions for her submissive will save herself a lot of time and avoid many annoyances such as unwished presences, unpleasant domestic noises, etc... There is only one drawback for heedless Mistresses : they may well forget in which spot of the house they have disconnected their submissive. Fortunately, this happens rarely...

3) Feminine deification

Such a progressive and necessary reification of males in a gynarchist system is the inevitable corollary of the natural deification of Women which will come alongside their ultimate rise to power.

Right from the beginings, Woman was deified. The Mother-Goddess is the first and only divinity that the human mind can conceive. A famous text by Simone de Beauvoir describes this clearly :

She is the queen of Heavens, she is represented as a dove; she is also the empress of Hell, she crawls out of Hell, she is symbolised as a snake. She is seen in mountains, in woods, on the sea, in springs. Everywhere she creates life; if she kills, she gives life again. She is whimsical, lustful, crual like Nature, at the same time propitious and fearsome, she reigns over all Aegid, Phrygia, Syria, Anatolia, over the entire western Asia. She is named Ishtar in Babylonia, Astarte by semitic peoples and Gea, Rhea or Cybele by Greeks; she can be found in Egypt under the appearance of Isis ; male deities are subordinate to Her.

Women in Gynarchy, as women, will of course have a tendency to self-deification, they will consider themselves as the driving Principle of the World and of Society. Lesbian love which, as we have seen, will soon become common, and then the general rule, will quickly make it easier to apprehend Female divinity. Males, as they will progressively be made to become things in the feminine society in which they will live, will also have a tendency to consider every woman, be she young or old, beautiful or ugly, as a Goddess to fear and worship devotedly. Their submission will thus be even more absolute and spiritually justified.

Gynarchy then will not only be a social and political system reaching perfection through human transcendence. Tied both to the terrestrial and the divine, it will be a universal Ideal.

CONCLUSION: GYNARCHY, A REALISTIC UTOPIA

Thus is Gynarchy a realistic, implementable utopia. Women will instate it in the course of the XXIst century, using the four references that we have briefly expounded here.

In the past, when the only references were Nature and the natural Authority of Mothers and thus of Women, Humankind lived in peace and harmony. The advent of patriarchy plunged the world into chaos and war. The rise to power of males was immediately followed by the instatement of injustice and misery. It is thus by returning to the sources of Nature, to the natural feminine power, that the human race can be regenerated. The World, born from Woman, must return humbly to Her to save itself.

Gynarchist philosophy is modern and pragmatic. It is more logical than any other system of thought, because it is eternal. The conception of the world induced by gynarchy is resolutely positive, turned towards a happy and peaceful future where even men will pick with happiness the sweet fruits of their submission from the magnificent tree of victorious, all-powerful feminity. Males, forever condemned to live in Women's shades, will find again in their abnegation their natural well-being as slaves deprived of any responsabilities.

The future, at last, is resolutely feminine. Men are more and more aware of their intrinsic deficiencies. Every passing day enlarges the gap between Woman and the male of the species, whose progressive degeneration becomes visible even to his own eyes. The political agenda offered by gynarchy for a social renewal is at the same time simple, revolutionary, full of practical sense, and far from any politician demagoguery.

No-one, deep in her/his heart, has ever been unaware that the future is gynarchist. What we have tried our best to do here was to promote this message in a written and militant way.

WOMEN ALL AROUND THE EARTH, UNITE !

The enslaving of males has begun.

Our reign is at last coming.

LONG LIVE GYNARCHY !

NOTES

1. Jan Jakob BACHOFEN (1815-1887), anthropologist and swiss lawyer, studied especially the passage from the primitive matriarchy to patriarchy, in *le Droit des mères*, 1861, and *Das Muterrecht* (Cf. Bibliothèque Nationale under ref. 8°R44461).

2. *Le Deuxième Sexe*, Paris, Gallimard, 1949.

3. Ibid.

4. Read *Les Femmes avant le patriarcat*, Paris, Payot, 1976, as well as *Le Féminisme ou la mort*, Paris, Pierre Horay, 1974.

5. Read *Amazones, guerrières et gaillardes*, Grenoble, Presses Universitaires de Grenoble, 1975.

6. The etymology of the world has been disputed. Its root means indeed, in ancient greek, breasts or teats. But the problem lies in the prefix : either it is the privative "a" (as the legend goes, the Amazons cut or compressed their right breasts in order to shoot better with their bows) or the augmentative "a" (the Amazons were also renowned for their significant beauty). Other etymologies have been suggested, such as : women with one veiled breast (only one visible breast), women eating flesh (non-vegetarian or cannibals), women with the belt (Ares's), women who love one another (lesbians), etc.

7. Libya, at the time of Diodorus, meant almost all Northern Africa. They could thus be located, without too much invention, in a land bordered to the north by the Hoggar mountains (where many matriarchal traces have been left, in particular within the Tuaregs where nobility is passed on through women), to the east by Cyrenaic, today's Lybia, all the way to Ethiopia, and to the south-west by the Gulf of Guinea (which borders former Dahomey where, at the turn of the twentieth century, an army of Amazons still held sway).

8. The numerous Abyssinian queens and the Amazons from Erythrea equally prove the historical reality of matriarchy in Ethiopia.

9. Heinrich Von Kleist balanced the myth in his *Penthésilea* (translated in french by Julien Gracq, Paris, José Corti, 1954). There, Achillus dies, a victim to the strength, the fiercery and the beauty of Penthesilea.

10. LE FEL, Marie-France, *Petit Dictionnaire historique et pratique de la domination et du sadisme des femmes*, Robert Laffont, Paris, 1981. p

11. Chevalier-Gheerbrant, *Dictionnaire des symboles*, Paris, Robert Laffont, p.28.

12. MARCIREAU, Jacques, *Histoire des rites sexuels*, Paris, Robert Laffont, 1971. p. 175.

13. This anecdote may explain why Alexander's immense conquests never included this small territory to the north-east of Asia Minor, at the foot of the Caucasus, the ancestral homeland of the Amazons.

14. See the *Grand Larousse du XIXe siècle*, the *Petit Dictionnaire* by Marie-France LE FEL (op.cit.) and the very beautiful novels by Marika MORESKI (*The Amazon*) and Christiane SINGER (*La Guerre des Filles*).

15. EAUBONNE, Françoise d', *Les Femmes avant le patriarcat*, op. cit. p. 70.

16. Society for Cutting Up Men.

17. Charlene DEERING, a new Amazon, also a lesbian, is the founder and Grand Priestess of the Femina-Society. Among her numerous writings, one can read these words : *I believe in Female Supremacy. All males must be at the feet of truly Dominant Women. Males are born to be slaves to Women, and this is the social order to come. Males are afraid of Female Superiority and this is why they try to condemn it wherever they can. Their worst crime has been to convince some women that males are superior ! I am happy to know that I am a Dominant Woman and that my slaves really desire to suffer for me and to learn thanks to my vast knowledge in the field of Female Supremacy* (FEMINA - the voice of Feminine Authority, nE5, printemps 92).

18. Cited by par Chevalier-Gheerbrant (op. cit.).

19. Op. cit. p . 50.

20. Some even qualify her as the "first modern Gynarchist". A very beautiful woman, she liked being sorrounded by favorites, who served her and whom she often treated badly. She had one fickle lover assassinated in front of her by her substitute. Perhaps because she was intrinsically lesbian, she never ceased to defend female pre-eminence.

21. And their figurehead husbands, of course ...

22. Simone de BEAUVOIR, op. cit. p. 180.

23. Called the Father Enfantin (1796-1864), a french engineer and a follower of Saint-Simons.

24. A feminist theoretician born in Minnesota in 1934, she took upon herself to fight men in the U.S.A. and denoucne their disgusting male chauvinism.

25. Movement for the castration of men.

26. On the benefits of sexual slavery for males, it is interesting to read a little book by Michel PLESSIER, Eloge de la servitude, published in 1994 by Spengler.

27. *Du bon usage des masochistes (About good Use of masochistic males)*, Paris, Diachroniques, 1987.

28. Heinrich Cornelius AGRIPPA VON NETTESHEIM, kabbalist medicine doctor and deutch philosoph wrting in latin (Cologn 1486 - Grenoble 1535). His *De occulta philosophia* (1529) and *De incertitudine et vanitate scientarium* (1527) got a

great success during century XVI. He was the doctor of François Ier's mother and the Charles Quint's historiograph.

29. Read about it the excellent essay of Simone de Beauvoir, *Le Deuxième sexe (The Second Gender)*.

30. See about the article WLASTA of *Petit dictionnaire historique et pratique de la domination et du sadisme des femmes*, by Marie-France LE FEL, and for theses that can consult it the *Grand Larousse du XIXe siècle* .

31. Thus Marie of Champagne, at the end of the 12th century, is demanding that Christian of Troyes, the hero of the Knight of the cart, ridicules himself in public for his beauty in the name of love.

32. Marguerite (1480-1530), daughter of the emperor Maximilian, was an admirable governor of the Netherlands and a fearsome politician. She concludes with the Duchess of Angoul me the famous Peace of Ladies and left a lot of autobiographical and poetical documents.

33. AGRIPPA, Heinrich Cornelius, *De la Supériorité des Femmes (About the Superiority of Women)*(1509), collection Théosophie Chrétienne , DERVY - BOOKS, Paris, 1986. (Text translated from the Latin, presented and annotated by Bernard DUBOURG, including philosophy).

34. In Hebrew: 'DM = Adam and 'DMH (adamah) = the earth. HWH (Hawwah) = Eve and HYH = to live.

35. The order of the divine Genesis is biblically and logically the following: mineral vegetable animal male Womyn.

36. Agrippa: op. cit. p.38.

37. Thus Salomon adoring Astarté and constructing a temple to each of 700 Womanly foreigners; as David raised Abiga l then Bethsabée to the highest functions; as, to Abraham himself, God orders: though Sarah, listen to Her voice (Genesis 21,12).

38. About the murderess treachery of Judith, Cornelius Agrippa says: Can one conceive of a more iniquitous project, more cruel treason, more insidious perfidy? And nevertheless it is to this gender of plots that the holy Handwriting awards its favors, its blessing, its eulogy, its encouragement's: everywhere, I repeat, the Bible grants the best reputation by far - to misdeeds of women rather than to the kindness of men." (op. cit. p.60.)

39. Let us not forget what the most recent Gynarchic research (the works of Valerie Solanas of S.C.U.M. in 1971) allows us to assert,: "The male is a biological accident; the (male) gene (y) is only an incomplete X gene (Female), an incomplete series of chromosomes. In others terms, the man is an unsuccessful woman, an itinerant miscarriage, a congenital runt. (...) virility is an organic deficiency, and men are the diminished..."

40. Aspasia, Dama, Gemina, Cathryn of Alexandria, etc.

41. In her Small historical and convenient dictionary of the domination and sadism of Women, Ms. Marie-France LE FEL, among the gallery of dominatrices that She presents to us, one finds more than a score of Lesbians!

42. For proof this extract from a work signed DORLES a wicked and Silly title where two Lesbians, having attached their male slaves to the ceiling, imagine them really hung : "We have a lot of pain to lull us, so much is delectable, the spectacle of these two naked men, suspended from the ceiling, above the bed where we are spread. I imagine Dick and Connie, hung by the neck, the pedantic language, « and I slip the hand between thighs of Paulette. My tender friend has without doubting the same thoughts as me, because Her hand searches my laces, slips on my stomach. I feel her fingers grind my clitoris. Our eyes are fixed on the two suspended slaves and our hands hurry, hurry and wet. Our stomachs have a jolt, our hands tense, our lips half-open to give sweet groans and our eyes close. The night envelopes our bodies snugly sunk in silky sheets under ridiculous and distended figures of our silent and submissive males."

43. To see this study subject and the indisputable conclusions of John Jacob BACHOFEN, Céline RENOOZ, Mrs. of PAINI, Simone of BEAUVOIR, Françoise of EAUBONNE, etc.

44. The male made its priests to wear dresses to and often required their chastity, to better convince the people of their quasi femininity. It made believe to children that Amazons were only mythological celebrities. Finally, it enslaves totally the Woman, declared himself "lord and master" or "head of the family" according to groups and periods, instituted even sometimes polygamy or, worse, the wearing of a vail on the face of Women, for the evident purpose of masking to eyes of the world his intrinsic male inferiority, particularly visible through the beauty of the face or the intelligence of the look of Women.

45. The "Sorceresses", US movement.

46. To see supra : Society for Cutting Up Men, "Association for the Castration of Men", an international movement created in the USA by the Lesbian Feminist Valerie SOLANAS.

47. " *The man is by nature a leech, an affective parasite, and no ethical reason justifies its life because nobody has the right to live at the expense of someone else. Similarly the life of humans rewards those animals for the sole reason that they are more evolved and endowed of a superior conscience. Similarly the life of Women has must excel that of men. Consequently to get rid of some men is a good and legitimate act that is all to the advantage of Women at the same time that it is an act of pity.* " Valerie SOLANAS, SCUM, 1967.

48. See the quotation of SCUM: *Remember that, by freezing, one can preserve the necessary sperm for a long time for the survival of humankind for thousands of years. Finally, these words, again, drawn from the SCUM Manifesto: The few men that will remain on the planet will have all the leisure to drag out their old puny days. They will be able to demolish themselves with drugs or to strut in rags or to watch the powerful Women as passive spectators, trying to live by proxy.*

49. One will read with interest the excellent and visionary poetic-philosophical novel of Monique WITTIG, *Les Guerillères* : "*They say, that they live, that they die, they don't have the power anymore.*" Op.cit. p.165.

50. Arguments of a "Femmocrate" of The Great war of the blues and the pinks, Norman spinrad : *The male's, physical characteristics are aggression and conquest. For him, aggression and sex are the same and it is the fuel of his masculinity. When a Sister caresses another Sister, there is neither penetration, nor dialectic rape between the hard and the soft, to give it and to take it. All gestures of their love become harmony, and the only force which appears is that which pushes the bodies, the spirits and the hearts to melt one into the other...*

51. Current technical progress now allows the most demanding of nymphomaniacs to have in Her handbag an erotic tool case replacing even the best trained male very well. Quote again Marie- France LE FEL : " *The erection, symbol of the male vitality, is often the target of the dominatrices who often is of saphiques and instincts Lesbian. The male virility in erection appears therefore, for these women, as a challenge or an insult to their supremacy and to their domination.* "

52. Marie-France LE FEL, again once : " *Most of the dominatrices recognize that they have no real sexual relations with their slaves. Many of them moreover being confirmed Lesbians, consider the idea of having sexual relations with them to be disgusting and that this would be too great an honor for them.* "

53. Origins of the man, the protohistory.

54. Prehistory to the historical period.

55. From century XVII.

56. First manifestations during century XX.

57. Probably from the middle of century XXI.

58. What is precisely the goal of this small book.

59. Cf. Gina Graham SCOTT, *The Feminine Domination*, Paris, Mérodack, 1987. " The fundamental principle is that the Woman has to be the object not only of erotic interest, but equally of adoration, because Her spiritual nature is superior that the man. " p.14.

60. *Society for Cutting Up Men*, see first chapter, second part.

61. One will note the convenient qualifier, confession of the militating goal of the author of this work.

62. And some historically inspired novels, or factual material, as *The Amazon, The Black Mistress*, etc.

63. *The Feminine Domination*, Paris, Robert Mérodack, 1987, and The Erotic Power, Paris, Robert Mérodack, 1986.

64. We think, with a lot others, that the fundamentalism, Muslim or catholic, is only the last desperate battle, of the obstructionist patriarchal world. The chauvinist play their last weapons and, as they have elsewhere always use blind violence and terrorism to combat the march of Feminine Power.

65. Paris, Mérodack, 1987.

66. Nature desires the institution of discipline, foundation of productive civilization and all coordinated human activity. Op. cit. p. 8.

67. *When I undertake to train a young animal human, I place it firmly under control. It has to understand that I am its MASTER, its friend. I tolerate no familiarity on its part. It speaks only when one addresses it and answers me "MADAM". In my presence, it remains upright and does not sit if I have not told it; even in this case it will without doubt sit cross-legged on the ground. It dresses or undresses on my order. It is whipped regularly and vigorously. It learns the virtues of humility and obedience.* Op. cit. p.9.

68. *Je dresse mon mari (I Train my Husband)*, Paris, Mérodack, 1989.

69. All three published by Robert Mérodack, Paris.

70. This last work, we will quote only some sentences the preface : *" I am called Astride and this work represents only a small part of my scientific and systematic program for the enslavement of all males. I intend to teach to women the most efficient manner to use their body to take the power, and I desire equally to scare men.*

" All men are excited by the idea of a "wicked" woman or "pervert". But, contrarily has an idea solidly established that associates automatically the masochism and the flagellation, perhaps the torture, I have discovered by experience that the masochistic fantasies most widespread in men consistently has him suffer and be humiliated by the body of the Woman.

" It results that a crack of a whip, an injection or a day in cage are less efficient than a slap, a tweak or an hour of suffocation under the hindquarters of a Woman.

My program aims therefore to use the greatest weakness of the man, namely the irresistible attraction that he feels for the Woman, Her appearance, Her voice, Her body and all of what She is normally capable. "

71. We prefer the word Teaching to that of Education, which seems us to connote a will to fashion opposite spirits to our principles. Remember that Gynarchy is the NATURAL government system of the world by the Woman and that it therefore invites to CONVERT and not to convince.

72. And it is well natural because these are the Students that profit mainly and in priority of our investments in " gray matter" and in material of teaching. More, the presence of boys avoids the considerable expense of service staff. It is natural that the expense on them is less.

73. Remember that the word GYNARCHY, means the Feminine POWER. We prefer to use, for its educational meaning, the word GYNOCRACY that designates rather the doctrine of the Feminine PRE-EMINENCE inside the Institution where the power is represented only by Teachers and the direction, of this power is partly exerted effectively by Students.

74. (To see figure #2) M = Master, S = Student, K = Knowledge. We will prefer however, for a best comprehension of our purpose, denominations M = Mistress, E = Student, A = Adjuvant, and S = Knowledge.

75. In the male courses, the coming and going is established only between the two intermediate Feminine Courses (adolescent Girls) or between extreme Courses (Young Women). Indeed, the adjuvant can perfect in THEORY only with the use of Students again to discover the utilization possibilities of the male (13-17 years), but, on the contrary, in the PRACTICE, its empirical knowledge acquisition demanded by the Gynarchie is easier by small girls spontaneous gynocratiquement (10-13 YEARS) or beside Womanly Youths at the end of Training and ready for entry into the university or active life (17-19 years).

76. Note 1 is attributed, after control, by the Mistress of the specific male Course. The note 2 is attributed in equal Council by Mistresses of the General Course, the Direction of the I.M.E.G., and the Delegated chosen of Students. As for notes 3 and 4, they are attributed alone by the Student - Holder of the adjuvant (this last being alone authorized to that and, to justify its note by an Observation in the File of the adjuvant). Thus, the notation and the possible sanctions of the auxiliary males are conditioned as much by scholastic homework as by individual service obligations.

77. The efficiency of an adjuvant, during the course, is measured by these three points very precisely:
- permanent and total silence,
- rapidity of execution of orders,
- legibility and exhaustiveness of notes manuscripts.

It is elsewhere on these same points that the Student -Holder notes its adjuvant each trimester.

78. The age limits on the admission of the adjutants to the I.M.E.G. is variable but one cannot nevertheless tolerate, beside our young Students, the presence of too old adults. For the former, the sole possibility of training remains in their participation in Sessions that our Mistresses and our last year Students organize often (in general for the purpose of finding the supplementary work to hand to these last!)

79. Indeed, if any Student - Holders at the I.M.E.G. has in priority of its successive adjutants (accredited during each of the cycles of its schooling) to exert the command and to study the psychology of the subordinated males, it can punctually, for specific works to the educative goal or entering within the framework convivial the community life (development of a magazine or theater piece or, a meal for a birthday, etc.), to ask that a certain number of other adjutants are placed temporarily under its orders (if it obtains nevertheless the preliminary agreement of the Director and that Students -Holders totally or partially deprived of their assistant).

80. Enter in these " technical competence" in all Feminine sciences allowing the access to the absolute power, social, professional and family, and the full exercise of the authority (arts of the seduction and domination, various punishment methods, mental and physical tortures, etc.).

81. The former, meanwhile, are occupied with the maintenance of the personal bedroom of their Student - Holder, placement in order of its business, sorting of clothes and dirty underclothes, complete cleaning of the bathroom, household...

82. Which are then in full athletic activity: swimming, volley ball, basketball, and tennis...

83.One will establish a corporal punishment gradation of type spanking by distinguishing those applied with naked hands, by the whip.

84. One will observe the isolation by - video link to one or several Students and the isolation cell is equipped with a video monitor connected to various cameras installed inside and to the exterior of buildings of the I.M.E.G. (Lounge and dining room of Students, Park, tennis courts, particular Chambers). To avoid all breach to the psyche of the sanctioned isolated, one will be able to leave in permanence to the former the vision on daily acts (meal, relaxation, athletic activity, perhaps sleep) of that to whom it has carried prejudice and that has wished its isolation during some days, that the former is or not its Student - Holder. The punished can thus live by proxy, the time of its isolation, the daily life of a Student.

85. To another I.M.E.G., in general abroad.

86. or subjection.

87. or subject.

88. or Sovereign.

89. The latin ergastulus : workshop where the Mistress encloses its slaves during the night. One speaks today of cowshed and, in U.S., "dungeon".

90. To read about this subject the Small Dictionary of Mrs. Marie-France LE FEL (op. cit.), to the slave article.

91.After the Enslavement, it is no longer necessary that the slave has a name. Alone its functional designation, or again a physical particularity, can henceforth largely suffice (flunkey, bootlicker, spittoon, castrated, etc.).

92. For this delicate and sensitive part of the training of the male, one will relate to the excellent work of Sophie DOMPIERRE, (op. cit.).

93. To see bibliography.

94. The terror of the resistant males opposing the revival of Gynarchy threatening their prerogatives has become such that they even try to assassinate Women that only try to be independent or cultivated. This blind violence released by Algerian male fundamentalists especially, is well the proof of the total disarray of these feeble chauvinists resisting the ascension of Women.

95. The area of the education having been processed supra (III, 1) and these of the army and the work, which feature in distinct chapters infra (IV, 2 and IV, 3).

96. Cf. supra (III, 1) p. 46.

97. Source I.N.S.E.E., 92 % of divorces take place in couples whose man has made its military service. 85 % take place in 5 years that follow it.

98. Among these young Women in charge of soldiers, sometimes of the same age as they but often undisciplined, will take care to see that the former execute to their chores to perfection particularly those that humiliate, so as to eradicate little by little all false male pride.

99. Due to concern for security, it will be well to always double systems of visual observation, to that even in case of failure, Surveillances could localize all male elements of whom they will have be in charge.

100. One will take care, to render more agreeable the work to males, who use suave feminine voices for the enumeration of orders to distribute.

101. To see under - chapter devoted to the Feminine week of three days.

102. Account held not, naturally, the possible ovine or bovine cattle heads.

103. One will not forget, in a purely hygienic goal, to distribute some erotic order (preferably saphiques to avoid all jealousy and bad assimilation) where the Feminine pleasure will be put well in evidence and exalted.

104. To see supra (VI, 1, 3)

105. It is proven: the males long submitted have more thoughts and sensations.

106. In the entirely gynarchized future world that we do wish, why not give the statute of "wall-dependant" to certain male slaves who could be yielded, in the real transactions of particular with particular, at the same time as the housing to which it affected and would be rivetted, like the sink, the bath-tub or the throne of the toilets? This measurement would have the advantage of having a slave always perfectly with the current of maintenance necessary to all the parts of housing in the course of transfer. Certain apartments could even take a certain real value thanks to the male which would be fixed there. I would like to welcome all women to my club, and have issues against men to talk about. Feminism is important, and should never be avoided. Go women.

107.Stool, lamp, table, hallstand, etc., furniture abilities for male are countless...
108.Op. cit. p. 121.

BIBLIOGRAPHY

THEORETICAL WORKS :

- AGRIPPA VON NETTESHEIM, Heinrich Cornelius, *De la Supériorité des femmes,* "opuscule traitant de la noblesse et de l'excellence du sexe féminin, et de sa supériorité sur le masculin", 1569, réédition : Paris, Dervy Livres, 1986.

- AKOUN, André (sous la direction de), *la Politique des Amazones,* article in *Mythes et croyances du monde entier,* t. 1 le Monde européen, Paris : Lidis-Brepols, 1985, p.71.

- ALBISTUR, Maïté & ARMOGATHE, Daniel, *Histoire du féminisme français du moyen-âge à nos jours,* Paris : Edition desFemmes, 1977, 508 p.

- ALMEIDA-TOPOR, Hélène d', *les Amazones,* Paris : Rochevigne, 1984, 188 p..

- ARBRANT, Aline d', *Petit guide de l'I.M.E.G.,* Gynarchy Club, Genève, 1993.

- ASTRIDE, *l'Art de l'étouffement,* Mérodack, Paris, 1988.

- ASTRIDE, *l'Art de l'excrétion,* Mérodack, Paris, 1989.

- ASTRIDE, *Puissance du jupon,* Mérodack, Paris, 1990.

- Athéna, Bulletin trimestriel, numéro spécial : *les Amazones,* Toulouse : Athéna Editions, n° double 51/52, octobre 1992, 96p.

- BACHOFEN, Johann Jakob, *Le Droit des Mères,* 1861.

- BERG, Jeanne de, *Cérémonies de Femmes,* Paris, Grasset.

- BEAUVOIR, Simone de, *Le Deuxième sexe,* Gallimard, Paris, 1949 et 1976 (réed. Coll. Folio Essais, n37).

- BERTRAND, Gabrielle, *Terres secrètes où règnent les femmes,* Livre contemporain, 1956.

- CHEVALIER, Alain et GHEERBRANT, Jean, *Dictionnaire des symboles,* Paris, Robert Laffont, 1969.

- CUVIER, Georges, *Le Règne animal distribué selon son organisation,* 1816-1817.

- DIODORE DE SICILE, *Histoire universelle,* Paris, Ed. de Bure, 1737-1891.

- DOMPIERRE, Sophie, *Je dresse mon mari,* Robert Mérodack, Paris, 1989.

- EAUBONNE, Françoise d', *Le féminisme ou la mort,* Paris : Pierre Horay, 1974, 276 p.

- EAUBONNE, Françoise d', *les Femmes avant le patriarcat,* Paris : Payot, 1976, 244 p.

- ELL, Lana, Introduction à *Capture et asservissement du mâle,* 1982.

- ENCYCLOPAEDIA UNIVERSALIS, nouvelle édition 1992.

- GHIRSHMAN, Roman, les *Cimmériens et leurs Amazones*, édition de Thérèse de Sonneville-David et Tania Ghirshman, Paris : Edition Recherche sur les Civilisations, 1983, 140 p.

- GRAHAM-SCOTT, Gini, *La Domination féminine*, Paris, Robert Mérodack, 1987.

- - , *le Pouvoir érotique*, Paris, Robert Mérodack, 1986.

- GRIMAL, Pierre, *Dictionnaire de la mythologie grecque et romaine*, Paris, P.U.F., 1951.

- GUYON, Abbé Claude Marie, *Histoire des Amazones anciennes et modernes*, Bruxelles : chez Jean Léonard, 1741, 210 p. ou Paris : chez Jean Villette, 1740.

- HERNANDEZ, Florence, *l'Etat de garce, Pourquoi et comment vivre comme une garce*, Paris : Albin Michel, 1995, 208 p.

- HUTIN, Serge, *Hommes et civilisations fantastiques*, Paris, J'ai Lu, 1971.

- LEDERER, Dr Wolfgang, *Gynophobia ou la Peur des femmes*, Trad. Monique Manin, Paris : Payot, 1970, 346 p

- LE FEL, Marie-France, *Petit dictionnaire historique et pratique de la domination et du sadisme des femmes*, Robert Laffont, Paris, 1981.

- LO DUCA, J.M., *Le Huitième sceau*, Paris, J.J. Pauvert.

- MARCIREAU, Jacques, *Histoire des rites sexuels*, Paris, Robert Laffont, 1971.

- PIGHETTI, Olivier, *Chez les animaux, la vie des mâles est un enfer !* in *Ça m'intéresse*, Paris, 1992.

- PLESSIER, Michel, *Eloge de la Servitude*, Paris, Spengler, 1994.

- SAMUEL, Pierre, *Amazones guerrières et gaillardes*, Grenoble, Complexe (Presses Universitaires de Grenoble), 1975.

- SANCHEZ, Jean-Pierre, *le Mythe des Amazones du Nouveau Monde*, Pamplona : Universidad de Navarra, Editions Reichenberger (coll. Acta Columbina), 1991, 66 p.

- SOLANAS, Valérie, *S.C.U.M., "le premier manifeste de la libération des femmes"*, présentation par Christiane Rochefort, Paris, Olympia, 1971.

- VIDAL-NAQUET, Pierre, *Esclavage et Gynécocratie in Le Chasseur noir, formes de pensées et formes de société dans le monde grec*, Paris : La Découverte, coll. textes à l'appui, 1991, 492 p.

- VILAR, Esther, *l'Homme subjugué*, Paris : Stock, 1972.

- WEBB, Wanda, Du *Bon usage des masochistes*, Mérodack, Paris, 1987.

INTERESTING TITLES OF WICH EVEN MALES COULD BENEFIT FROM :

a) detectives/adventures

- BEHM, Marc, *la Reine de la nuit*, Paris : Rivages, 1992, 266 p.

- BRICE, Michel, *La Secte des Amazones*, Paris, Plon, 1979.

- BRICE, Michel, *les Maîtresses-Femmes de Saint-Tropez*, Paris, Plon.
- CHASE, James-Hadley, *Eva*, Paris, Gallimard.
- CONNERS, Bernard F., *la Dernière danse*, Paris, Livre de poche.
- DARD, Frédéric, *le Maître de plaisir*, Paris, Fleuve noir.
- LANE, Ernie, *l'Ange du Diable*, Paris : Bellevue (coll. Le Roman de choc n°8), 1973, 192 p.
- LAY, André, *Vallespi chez les Amazones*, Paris : Fleuve Noir, coll. Spécial-Police n° 1168, 1975, 240 p.
- MAC BAIN, Ed, *Kiss*, Paris, Presses de la Cité, 1994.
- MAC BAIN, Ed, *Poissons d'avril*, Paris, Presses de la Cité, 1995.
- MANCHETTE, Jean-Patrick, *Fatale*, Paris : Gallimard, 1977, 192 p.
- ROHMER, Sax, *Nude in mink*, trad. Alex Stoya : *Nue sous un manteau de vison*, Paris : Del Duca/Les Editions Mondiales, coll. le Basilic rouge n° 10, 1951, 224 p.
- SCOPPETTONE, Sandra, *Everything you have is mine*, trad. de Christophe Claro, Tout ce qui est à toi..., Paris : Fleuve Noir, 1995, 416 p.
  b) science fiction.
- BLOCH, Robert, *Matriarchie*, Verviers, Marabout, 1975.
- BRADLEY, Marion Zimmer, *Free Amazons of Darkover*, Gordon Mc Gill, 1995, trad. de Simone Hilling : *les Amazones libres*, Paris : Phébus, 1990, reed. Presses Pocket n°5564, 1995, 320 p.
- BRADLEY, Marion Zimmer, *la Maison des Amazones*, trad. de Simone Hilling , Paris : Presses Pocket n°5510, 1993, 448 p.
- CHANBERT, Daniel-Yves, *Les Sirènes de Lusinia*, Paris, Albin-Michel, 1974.
- GUNN, James, *le Misogyne*, in *Grande Anthologie de la science-fiction, histoires à rebours*, Paris : Le Livre de poche, 1976, pp. 55-68.
- MAZARIN, Jean, *Libérez l'homme !*, Paris, Fleuve noir, 1979.
- MERLE, Robert, *Les Hommes protégés*, Paris, Gallimard, 1974.
- SPINRAD, Norman, *La Grande guerre des Bleus et des Roses*, Paris, Robert Laffont, 1980.
- VEILLOT, Claude, Misandra, Paris, J'ai Lu, 1974.
- WEST, John Anthony, *le Gregory de Gladys*, in *Grande Anthologie de la science-fiction, histoires à rebours*, Paris : Le Livre de poche, 1976, pp. 21-31.
  c) classical and historical, theater.
- BERG, Jeanne de, *Cérémonies de femmes*, Paris : Grasset.
- CHOLODENKO, Marc, *Histoire de Vivant Lannon*, Paris, Folio.
- KLEIST, Heinrich Von, *Penthésilée*, 1811.
- MORESKI, Marika, *L'Amazone*, Paris, Concorde, 1979.
- RAYNAL, Henri, *Aux pieds d'Omphale*, Paris, J.J. Pauvert.

- SACHER-MASOCH, Léopold, *La Vénus aux fourrures*, préface de Gilles DELEUZE, Paris, 10/18.

- SACHER-MASOCH, Léopold, *Fouets et fourrures*, Paris, Le Castor astral, 1995.

- SINGER, Christiane, *La Guerre des filles*, Paris, Albin-Michel, 1981.

- SOURDINE, Thomas, *la Démolition*, Halévy, Paris 1970.

- WHIPPLE, Gay, *Sadie Maize*, Trad. de José Pitrangeli : *Sadie... que ça dit...*, intr. de Niels Lindströmm, Kalmthout-Anvers : Walter Beckers, 1970, 300 p.

- WITTIG, Monique, *Les Guérillères*, Paris, Les Editions de Minuit, 1969.

d) comics.

- Anonyme, *les Dévoreuses d'hommes*, in *Jungla*, mensuel n° 32, Paris : Elvipress, mars 1973.

- Anonyme, *les Bêtes*, in *Psycho*, n° 1, Paris : Les Editions de Poche, 1972, pp. 39-42.

- Anonyme, *l'Île des orgies*, in *Jungla*, mensuel n° 6, Paris : Elvipress, 1970.

- BELLAMY, Garth, *la chasse à l'homme,* in *Charlie* mensuel, n°122, Paris : Charlie, 1979, pp. 82-98.

- BULANADI, Danny, & ROSTLER, William, *Tarzan, au pays des Amazones*, d'après Edgar Rice Burroughs, in *Tarzan*, n° 54, Paris : Sagédition, 1978, pp. 35-49.

- CORIA-VERNES, *Un parfum d'Ylang-Ylang* (Bob Morane), Bruxelles, Le Lombard, 1995.

- CUVELIER-VAN HAMME, *Epoxy*, Paris, Horus, 1977.

- DIONNET, J.P. et POIVET,R., TIRIEL, *Héritier d'un monde*, Paris, Nathan, 1975.

- ENEG, *Kageena*, in *les Hordes de Phobos*, n°1, Paris : Futuropolis, 1974, pp. 27-31.

- GARCIA, Luis, & MC GREGOR, Donald F., *les Prêtresses de Diane*, in Vampirella, n°6, New York : Warren Publishing Co, & Paris : Publicness, 1971, pp. 23-34.

- GRAHAM, Billy, & FOX, Gardner, *Amazonia, l'œil d'Oisirios*, in *Vampirella*, n°8, New York : Warren Publishing Co, & Paris : Publicness, 1971, pp. 56-63.

- HOPPER, J.H., *Madame*, Vitry, Comix Trading France, 1990.

- HUGDEBERT, *Irina*, Vitry, Loempia, 1995.

- JERONATON, *Amazones*, in *Métal Hurlant* n92 à 97, Paris, Les Humanoïdes Associés, 1983.

- PELLAERT, G. et BARTIER, P., Les Aventures de Jodelle, Paris, Eric Losfeld, 1966.

- ROBBINS, Trina, *Montezuma's revenge*, in *Girl fight comics*, #2, Berkeley : Print Mint, 1974, pp. 1-10.

- ROSINSKI & VAN HAMME, *le Grand Pouvoir du Chninkel*, Tournai : Casterman, 1988, 168 p.
- SERAFÍN, *Carmen, Underground II*, Madrid : Gisa Ediciones S.A., 1975, 104 p.
- STURGEON, Fulbert, The *Amazons on the field of honnor*, in *Amazon comics*, San Francisco : Rip of Press, 1972.
- WARD, Bill et KEISTER, Bart, *la Saga des soeurs Chevrotine*, Paris, Pink Star, 1989.
e) filmography.
- ADAMSON, Al, *The Female bunch*, USA, 1971 (with Russ Tamblyn, Jenifer Bishop).
- ALMODOVAR, Pedro, *Matador*, Espagne, 1985, (with Asumpta Serna).
- BAKER, Roy Ward, *Moon zero two*, G.B., 1970 (with James Olson, Catherine Schell).
- BERNDS, Edward, *Queen of outer space*, USA, 1958 (with Zsa Zsa Gabor, Eric Fleming).
- BLIER, Bertrand, *Calmos*, France, 1976 (with J. Rochefort, J.P. Marielle, B. Blier).
- CARRERAS, Michaël, *Prehistoric women*, USA, 1966 (with Martine Beswick).
- CHU, Yin Ping, *les Sept Magnifiques*, Japon, 1984 (with Venus Lin).
- CIMBER, Matt, Hundra, USA, 1990 (with Laurene Landon).
- DAHL, John, *Last seduction*, USA, 1993 (with Linda Fiorentino, Peter Greg).
- DALLAMANO, Massimo, *Venus im pelz*), 1969 (with Laura Antonelli).
- DANTE, Joe, (et Carl GOTTLIEB, John LANDIS) *Amazon women on the moon*, USA, 1987 (with Ralph Bellamy, Rosanna Arquette, Michelle Pjeiffer).
- DAY, Robert, *She*, USA, 1964 (with Ursula Andress et Peter Cushing).
- DEIN, Edward, *Leech Woman*, USA, 1960 (with Coleen Gray).
- DEMME, Jonathan, *Cinq Femmes à abattre*, USA, 1974 (with Juanita Brown, Barbara Steele, a "Renegade Women Co-productions").
- EDMONDS, Don, *Harem*, USA, 1975, (with Dyanne Thorne).
- FELLINI, Federico, *la Cité des femmes*, Italie, 1979 (with Anna Prucnal et Marcello Mastroianni).
- FRANCISCI, Pietro, *Hercule et la reine de Lydie*, 1958 (with Christopher Reeves, Sylvia Koscina).
- FRANCO, Jesus, *la Ciudad sin hombres*, Espagne, 1970 (with Shirley Eaton).
- GANTILLON, Bruno, *Servante et maîtresse*, 1976 (with Andréa Ferreol, Victor Lanoux).
- GARTNER, James, *Golden Temple Amazons*, USA, 1986 (with Joan Virly).

- GRANIER-DEFERRE, Pierre, *Cours privé*, France, 1986 (with Elisabeth Bourgine, Michel Aumont).
- GLASER, Paul-Michaël, *Amazons*, USA, 1984 (with Tamara Dobson, Madeleine Stowe).
- GUEST, Christopher, *Attack of the 50 feet woman*, USA, 1995, (with Daryl Hannah).
- HELGENBERGER, Marc, *Mutante*, USA 1995, (with natacha Henstridge).
- HILTON, Arthur, *les Femmes-chats de la Lune*, USA, 1953.
- JURAN, Nathan, *Attack of the 50 feet woman*, USA, 1958.
- JUSTMAN, Robert, *Planet Earth*, (with J. Saxon, D. Muldaur).
- KAPLAN, Jonathan, *Bad girls*, USA, 1994, (with Madeleine Stowe, Andy McDowell...)
- LAFLEUR, Jean, *She-wolf of the SS*, USA, 1974 (with Dyanne Thorne).
- LAMONT, Charles, *Abbott and Costello go to Mars*, USA, 1953.
- LAWTON-, J.F., *Cannibal Women in the avocado jungle*, USA, 1988 (with Shannon Tweed, Adrienne Barbeau)
- LEONVIOLA, Antonio, *les Gladiatrices*, 1962.
- LOSEY, Joseph, *Eva*, USA, 1962 (with Jeanne Moreau).
- LOSEY, Joseph, *Modesty Blaise*, USA, 1965 (with Monica Vitti, Rossella Falk).
- MEDAK, Peter, *Romeo is bleeding*, USA, 1958 (with Lena Olin, Gary Oldman, Juliette Lewis).
- NEGRONI, Baltassare, *l'Amazzone mascherata*, Italie, 1914, (with Francesca Bertini).
- NESHER, Avi, *She*, USA, 1985 (with Sandahl Bergman).
- NEUMANN, Kurt, *Tarzan and the Amazons*, 1945 (with Brenda Joyce, Johnny Weissmuller).
- PETRI, Elio, *la Decima Vittima*, 1966 (with Ursula Andress, Marcello Mastroiani).
- REITMAN, Ivan, *Cannibal Girls*, 1973 (with Andrea Martin).
- ROTH, Cy, *Fire maidens from outer space*, G.B. 1956.
- SALA, Vittorio, *la Reine des Amazones*, 1960 (with Gianna Maria Canale).
- SCHROEDER, Barbet, *Maîtresse*, 1976 (with Bulle Ogier, Gérard Depardieu).
- SCOTT, Ridley, *Thelma et Louise*, USA, 1990 (with Susan Sarandon et Geena Davis).
- SIODMACK, Kurt, *Love slaves of Amazons*, 1958 (with Don Taylor).
- SJÖBERG, Alf, *Mademoiselle Julie*, Suède, 1951 (with Anita Björk).
- THOMAS, Ralph, *Deadlier than the male*, G.B., 1967, (with Syla Koscina, Suzanna Leigh, Richard Johnson).

- VERHOEVEN, Paul, *Basic instinct*, USA, 1992 (with Sharon Stone, Michael Douglas).
- WORTH, david, *Angel of fury*, USA, 1994, (with Cynthia Rothrock).
- WEISS, Don, *Amazones*, USA, (with Elaine Stewart, John Derek).
- WOLCOTT, James L., *Wild women of Wongo*, (with Jean Hawkshaw).
- WORTMANN, Sönke, *Allein unter frauen*, Allemagne, 1994 (with Jennifer Nitsch, Thomas Heinze).

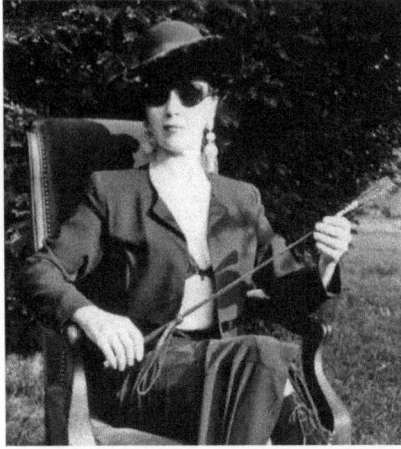

About the Author

Aline d'Arbrant (1952-2017) is the foundress of the gynarchist movement.

It is the *SCUM Manifesto* which will inspire her essay *The Gynarchy* which will in turn become an international best seller.

Eighteen short stories and a dozen novels will follow, all describing women, couples, families, societies or gynarchist worlds.

Aline d'Arbrant also wanted to promote certain famous or forgotten titles: first some short stories by **Léopold Sacher-Masoch**, then her famous Venus in fur, of which she will make an amusing gynarchic reading that will conclude with humor her Letters from Saphine to Wanda, then **Bérangère**'s novel *Josiane and her slave*.

Aline d'Arbrant is the foundress of the **Gynarchy International** association under french law (law of 1901) which aims to "*make known the ideas and the gynarchist theories, as described in particular in the works of Aline d'Arbrant, in France, in Europe and throughout the world; to act at all levels to assert the exclusively non-venal gynarchist aspirations and, in general, to promote a preponderant position of women in the private, social and political life of all countries; develop a politico-social project based on female predominance and capable of responding to the challenges facing the world today; contribute to the creation of gynarchist* *micro-societies that can serve as models of society for states and humanity whole; to federate all the organizations which, across the planet, are dedicated to female supremacy and to women's access to positions of political, industrial and financial power; to fund and organize events, meetings, exhibitions relating to its objects; encourage the creation of think tanks to propose solutions to common gynarchist problems of interest to members; manage a civil real estate company whose buildings and land, owned or rented, could be used by its members in compliance with the objects of the association and its possible internal regulations."*

Read more at gynarchy.org.

Milton Keynes UK
Ingram Content Group UK Ltd.
UKHW011324180923
428900UK00001B/31

9 798215 248904